Lea Stening

HEALTHY KIDS, HAPPY LIVES

Disclaimer

This booklet provides a general summary of the subject matter covered; it is not a substitute for informed professional advice. People affected by weight concerns (including family/whanau and others who provide support) should seek professional advice about their individual situation. Lea Stening Health is not liable for any error or omission in this publication, as a result of negligence or otherwise.

Copyright

Copyright © 2017 by Lea Stening

All rights reserved. No part of this publication text may be uploaded or posted online without the prior written permission of the publisher.

For permission requests, write to the publisher, addressed "Attention: Permissions Request," to nutrition@leastening.com.

A catalogue record for this book is available from the National Library of New Zealand.

Table of contents

Introduction — 6

It's fun to watch children growing — 7

Eight tips to manage growth — 10

What does being healthy mean? — 14

Life takes a lot of energy — 18

Ten ways to stay healthy — 25

Healthy baseline meal plan — 42

Shopping tips — 50

Reading food labels — 51

Food apps — 58

Have fun with food — 59

Finally — 60

Recipes — 61

Additional Recipes and Resources — 80

About the Author — 81

Introduction

It's a family affair

Obesity is a global problem. In New Zealand, 33% of children and 65% of adults are overweight or obese. The New Zealand population now rates as the third fattest in the OECD after USA and Mexico.

There are also 240,000 people with diabetes living in New Zealand, with a growing contingent of those with Type 2 diabetes. This type used to only affect adults over 40 years of age and, rarely, children under 18 years. Now obesity is causing ten-year-olds to develop diabetes. Somehow we are going astray.

We all want our children to live healthy and happy lives and to reach their full potential. This book is designed as a simple resource to help you and your family, wherever you are, to build sustainable energy by developing a healthy lifestyle and body weight, so you can power through your day with enough energy left over to enjoy each other.

Throughout this book, you will find **bit.ly** links to a variety of recent articles, written and posted by Lea on her website, designed to offer you a deeper understanding of nutrition issues, practical tips, and advice. (Bit.ly links are short web addresses that are easier to type into your browser and will take you to the original online article.)

In recognition that people now travel to places around the world and where food regulations differ, references have also been given to resources available on these subjects in New Zealand, Australia, UK, China and USA.

If you have any concerns regarding your child's health, talk to your doctor and local registered dietitian.

It's fun to watch children growing

The measurement of a child's growth in height and weight can be a good place to start when looking at their overall health. While growth rates are very individual, children usually sustain a steady growth rate between the ages of two to 10 years old.

A final growth spurts begins at puberty, which appears around the ages of 10 to 14 years in girls and 12 to 16 years in boys.

How do you measure a child's growth rate?

There are three main methods useful for monitoring children's growth.

Waist circumference measurements

This is a useful way of tracking changes in children under 12 years.

World Health Organisation Standard Growth Charts

These charts are useful for tracking the proportions of children's growth. The 50th percentile line is the average progression for age. Height normally exceeds weight, particularly for boys during rapid periods of growth. If your child's height is not progressing, or weight exceeds height into the 85th to 97th percentile or beyond, this is an important topic to discuss with your doctor or paediatric dietitian.

You can download these charts to use at home:

> Weight-for-age (5–10 years): Girls (bit.ly/2jOnQxJ) [PDF] - Boys (bit.ly/2jAjYDq) [PDF]
> Height-for-age (5–19 years): Girls (bit.ly/2jO9rSt) [PDF] - Boys (bit.ly/2iM74O0) [PDF]

These charts are also available in imperial mesasurement if you prefer:

> Stature-for-age and Weight-for-age (2–20 years): Girls (bit.ly/2iM1ueQ) [PDF] - Boys (bit.ly/2jAkK3n)[PDF]

Body Mass Index (BMI)

This is a useful tool to relate weight to height for adults (18 years and over). BMI is calculated by dividing weight (body mass) in kilograms or pounds by the square of the body height in metres or inches. If using pounds and inches, multiply the result by 703.

Diagram 1: BMI calculation

$$BMI_{\text{(metric)}} = \frac{mass\ (kg)}{(height\ (m))^2} \qquad BMI_{\text{(imperial)}} = \frac{mass\ (lb)}{(height\ (in))^2} \times 703$$

A healthy BMI is 18.5–24.99, overweight is >25, and obese is > 30.

Either side of this healthy BMI range problems can occur. As BMI drops <18.5 there is a greater risk of bone thinning, fatigue and immune insufficiency and as BMI increases towards 25 the risk of diabetes, heart disease and obesity rises.

The World Health Organisation (WHO) recommends using these same BMI cut-off points for all adults irrespective of their age, sex or ethnicity.

Child Growth Reference Charts

Since the BMI of children rapidly changes as they mature, and growth rates differ between boys and girls, this increases the difficulty of BMI assessment for children.

Instead of using the fixed BMI thresholds (designed for adults), these charts are compared to a reference group of children. This is known as a 'child growth reference'. This shows a pattern of growth and average BMI at a particular age and the percentage of variation.

Diagram 2: Peter's BMI calculation

Peter is 10 years old, weighs 44kg (97lbs) and his height is 1.45m (57in). He has a BMI of 21.

$$\text{Peter's BMI (metric)} = \frac{44}{1.45^2} = 21.0 \qquad \text{Peter's BMI (imperial)} = \frac{97}{57^2} \times 703 = 21.0$$

While a BMI of 21 would be healthy for an adult (a healthy BMI range is 18.5–24.99), the children's BMI chart below puts Peter on the 97th BMI range for his age. Peter's BMI may need monitoring by his doctor or dietitian.

You can download these charts to use at home:

> Body mass index-for-age (5–19 years): Girls (bit.ly/2k6iPUP) [PDF] - Boys (bit.ly/2jAnhdK) [PDF]

Or in imperial measurement if you prefer:

> Body mass index-for-age (2–20 years): Girls (bit.ly/2jOrpE7) [PDF] - Boys (bit.ly/2jqHj89) [PDF]

Eight tips to manage growth

If you have concerns about your child's weight, these few tips might be of help:

1. Avoid negative talk

Studies show that teasing, bullying, and name-calling regarding weight makes matters worse. You can't 'shame your child slimmer'; these sorts of comments will only make a child feel anxious and depressed, and lead to poor self-esteem.

Also avoid making negative comments about your own weight or other people's efforts at weight loss. Especially avoid encouraging the use of radical fad diets or dietary supplements.

2. Focus on and nurture the talents of your child

When a child can see that any achievement in life (e.g. academic or sporting success, development of computer skills or artistic talents, etc.) takes hard work but is attainable, this builds their self-esteem. These scenarios also raise the possibility that the same amount of effort, when focused on improving health, can also make weight and fitness goals achievable.

3. Focus on healthy eating as a source of energy for reaching goals

If a child loves to play a particular sport, encouraging healthy eating as an important part of their sport's nutritional goals is likely to prove more empowering than a negative message.

For instance, saying that "healthy eating provides specific energy and nutrients for sport performance" might be more encouraging to your child than saying "eating junk food results in heart disease or bone loss later in life." If the child is more inclined toward art, music, or academics, the same strategy can also apply.

4. Make home an easy place for health and fitness

This could include buying fresher, healthier food. For instance, parents can bring home more fruit and vegetables as snack items, or start a vegetable garden. As parents, you can also model behaviours for your children to emulate, such as snacking on vegetable sticks with hummus rather than crisps, going for a walk after dinner, and deciding not to keep a television in the bedroom.

As parents are the gatekeepers of food, and provide most of the cues for physical activity and small screen recreation, it is important for you to take part in any family intervention.

5. Switch from negative food messages to a positive approach

Rather than focusing on media reports of quick weight loss diets or formulas, or joining into the good food/junk food debate, focus instead on healthy food as a source of nutrients that build stronger, fitter bodies. Keep a positive attitude by encouraging your children to talk about their feelings, showing genuine concern and notice when they make an effort to make healthier food choices and to exercise.

6. Learn about the quantities of food needed for growth and development

For both you and your children, it is important to understand both the correct quantities and portion sizes of foods that stop hunger. Encourage children to try a wide range of different foods as they learn to prepare simple meals and snacks that everyone can enjoy.

7. Provide a supportive environment

Promote lots of talking and even more listening in your home environment. Research shows that shared family meal times can protect against disordered eating behaviours, providing an important time for children to share experiences of the day and connect with one another. Avoid unnecessary distractions by turning off the television during meal times.

8. Seek professional help

Existing evidence supports the view that childhood programs which address weight issues (excess weight gain or loss) are not associated with psychological harm. Of course, the intervention should focus on a healthy diet, physical activity, and behavioural management techniques: problem solving, goal setting, managing change, self-monitoring, and healthy thinking (regarding food, the body, and relapse prevention).

The program should last for a minimum of 12 weeks, include parental involvement, and provide medical supervision.

Concerned about your child?

If your concerns are growing, take action now:

> See your doctor to check your child's health and growth rate.
> Start thinking about ways to increase exercise as a family.
> Talk to your wider family about the need to co-operate with healthier eating when you visit them (Ref: Grandparents can help fight childhood obesity - bit.ly/2iM9tZ9).
> Tune into your parenting style to see if there are elements from your own upbringing that are affecting/helping how you manage your children now (Ref: Tune into your parenting style for better child health - bit.ly/2k36nkH).
> Make an appointment if you would like to see your local paediatric dietitian, or contact Lea for an online Skype appointment by emailing her at nutrition@leastening.com.

Further reading

For additional information, consider reviewing these resources:

> Clinical Guidelines for Weight Management in NZ children and Young People (bit.ly/2kYIV8E)
> Changing our weight talk may bring better health (bit.ly/2jAsdPR)
> Overcome misconceptions about weight for better family health (bit.ly/2jBDY8b)
> Does your diet tick all the boxes? (bit.ly/2jObd5J)

What does being healthy mean?

As a parent, if you want to help your child attain better health, a good place to start could mean talking about what being 'healthy' means to them.

We hear a lot today about the importance of diet and exercise through the media, television shows, and magazines. While everyone seems to be talking about good physical health, what about mental health? Doesn't being healthy also mean feeling safe and connected with friends and family, having work to do, feeling valued and loved, being happy, and learning new things?

Many people see their diet as a cloud that hangs over them. Often it spoils their fun because they worry about their weight, feel tired, frustrated, and maybe even get depressed.

Your diet isn't you! Ideally, a 'healthy diet' (i.e. the sum of what you eat per day) should instead form the hub of the wheel to your life, giving you the energy and power to do the things you want to do as well as the things that you have to do each day.

We use this simple concept as part of our weight control programs (bit.ly/2klVbms) and find it really helps families to better balance their time and energy.

Do you feel your diet offers balance to your life? Is it giving you the energy to enjoy each day? What could you change?

Figure 1: The Healthy Diet Hub of Life

Ideally a 'healthy diet' (i.e. the sum of what you eat per day) should form the hub of the wheel to your life giving you energy and power each day.

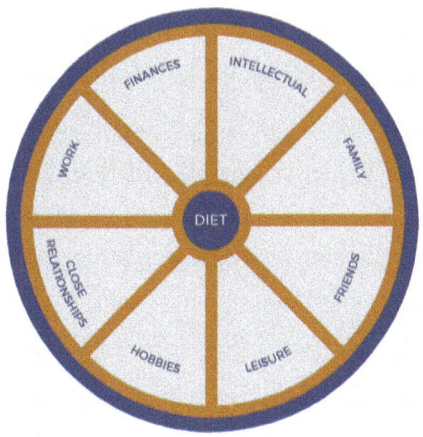

Try this exercise

Using a scale of 1 to 10 (10: Good, 1: Needs work), write down how happy you are with the time you spend beside each section of the wheel portrayed above. What time could you re-allocate, e.g. if you want more money, can you do more work? If you want to get more fit, can you combine an activity with seeing your friends, perhaps running or going on a bike ride together?

Do you have any unhelpful lifestyle habits?

Consider any habits that could be affecting your health and food intake: sleeping in, skipping meals, working too late, binge eating or drinking late at night, over-celebrating, eating in front of TV, etc. What could you change first?

Do other people influence what you eat and drink?

For example, do you eat or drink differently with family and friends than when you are alone? Do you pick at food leftovers? Do you tend to have more takeaway or snack foods when you are with certain people? Who supports you in being the healthiest version of you, and can you spend more time with them?

Do you eat for non-hungry reasons?

Do you eat for reasons other than hunger, such as stress relief for an emotional state – when you are feeling lonely, upset, or bored? Make a list of other things that you could do instead: go for a run, listen to music, talk to your parents or a friend about your day, etc. Maybe you could take up a hobby like photography or design.

Record your food and fluid intake for a week

Record your food and fluid intake for a week; perhaps also record your exercise and hours of sleep. Then read this book and think about a few things that you could change.

Try the Five Ways to Well-being

As well as encouraging your children to think more about their eating habits, also get them to tune into the positive things going on around them.

These five simple strategies from the NZ Mental Health Foundation might help them to do this:

1. **Connect**: Talk and listen; be there and feel connected to others.
2. **Give**: Your time, your words, your presence
3. **Take notice**: Remember the simple things that give you joy.

4. **Keep learning**: Embrace new experiences, see opportunities, and surprise yourself by trying new things.
5. **Be active**: Do what you can, enjoy what you do, move your mood forward.

Further reading

> Five Ways to Wellbeing: A best practice guide (bit.ly/2jOBjrp) [PDF]

Life takes a lot of energy

It takes a lot of energy to grow, exercise, play sport, learn, cope with change, and create. This energy comes from, you guessed it... food!

Defining a healthy diet

Around the world, health authorities have developed food models to teach people about food groups and to offer guidance on the proportions of foods required in order to achieve good health through better nutrition.

What do these food models have in common?

> - Put simply, they encourage us to eat most from the food groups that grow from the ground (i.e breads, cereals, fruits, and vegetables). These foods give us **carbohydrates** (i.e starches and sugars) for energy and dietary fibre, which is important for the health of our digestive tract, bowels, and weight management.
> - They recognise the importance of animal foods such as meat, fish, poultry, milk and milk products, as well as tofu, peas, and beans for **protein,** as this helps us to grow and replace tissue.
> - Recognition is also given to **fats** and oils as in small amounts; these are important for brain and nerve development.
> - **Fluids** help to regulate body temperature, distribute energy and nutrients around our body, and remove waste. We are encouraged to drink more low-fat milk and water and to limit alcohol intake.

Figure 2: Nutrition education around the world

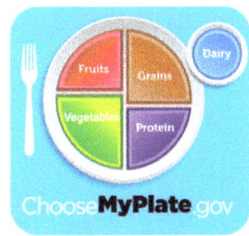

MyPlate — U.S. Department of Agriculture
(bit.ly/2ljPd3M)

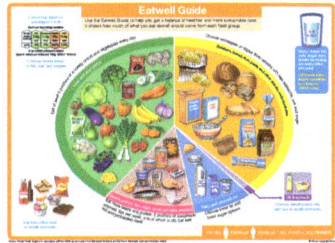

The Eatwell Guide — Public Health England
(bit.ly/2kHOWdh)

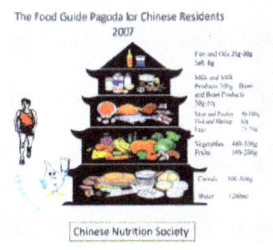

The Food Guide Pagoda 2007 — Chinese
Nutrition Society (bit.ly/2kgNj2X)

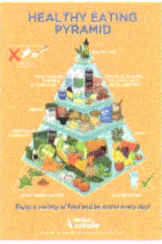

The Healthy Eating Pyramid — Nutrition
Australia (bit.ly/2kgJqL4)

› In the guidelines that accompany these food models, there is also the encouragement to limit added sugar and salt, and to engage in physical activity and exercise.

› Extra dietary supplements, vitamins, and minerals are not recommended unless directed by your doctor.

What is energy?

When foods and certain fluids are consumed, they release heat. This heat can be measured as kilocalories (kcals). The metric term for this is kilojoules (kJ).

1 kilocalorie = 4.18 kilojoules

Table 1: The energy content of food groups

Food group	Kilocalories/kilojoules per gram
Protein e.g. meat, fish, eggs, cheese	4/17
Carbohydrate e.g. bread, cereals, fruit, vegetables	4/17
Fat e.g. butter, margarine & oils	9/37
Alcohol (not recommended for children)	7/29

As you can see, alcohol and fat carry nearly twice as many calories as proteins and carbohydrates; this is just one reason why the intake of alcohol and fat should be limited for weight management and good health.

How much energy do we need each day?

The amount of energy required to keep a child alive and healthy is known as the Basal Metabolic Rate (BMR). This rate varies according to the child's body size, body composition, age, gender, and nutritional state. Added to this is your child's need for growth and physical activity.

To prevent chronic disease, it is generally recommended that energy should come proportionally from the following food groups:

> **Protein:** 10-25%
> **Fat:** 20-35%
> **Carbohydrate:** 45-65%

For a child 5 to 10 years, growing at a steady rate, it would be acceptable to have an average of 15% protein, 30% fat, and 55% carbohydrate. In comparison, an athletic adolescent boy may need 15% protein, 25% fat, and 60% cabohydrate. A dietitian can assist you to determine your children's energy needs as they grow and exercise.

Also see "Table 2: The number of servings of food groups required by children of different age groups." All of this growing uses energy, so it is not surprising that children often complain of feeling hungry.

Signs of hunger

Signs of hunger vary from one person to another. Not all of us feel a sinking sensation in our stomach when we run out of food and our blood sugar (fuel level) starts falling. Some people experience sugar cravings, some may start shaking, others may notice feelings of fatigue and changes in mood and attentiveness. Feelings of stress and agitation may also increase as people struggle to maintain their levels of concentration and physical performance.

To avoid feeling **hungry,** and maintain blood sugar levels, it helps to eat the **right foods,** in the **right amount** at the **right time.**

The 'right' amount depends on a person's age, growth rate, activity level, culture, etc. However, broadly speaking, understanding how to maintain an even blood glucose level can really help to sustain energy levels to power through the day.

Timing is everything

Have you ever noticed that after eating, even healthy food, you feel full at the time and then get hungry after an hour or two? When this cycle occurs, you may be more likely to snack on less healthy food.

The combination of foods and the speed at which these foods are digested determines how full we feel, and how far the energy released from these foods will drive us throughout our day.

As foods digest, they release their energy at different rates of time:

> **Carbohydrate foods**: Energy release between ½–2 hours (depending on their glycaemic index ref "The Glycaemic Index")
> **Protein foods**: Digest over 3–4 hours
> **Fats and oils:** Digest over 4–5 hours

Although there may be slight individual variation, assuming in the diagram below that breakfast is taken at 7 a.m., if we were to just eat foods containing carbohydrates (e.g. fruit and cereal) within 30 minutes to two hours, our blood sugar levels would start to fall.

However, if at 7 a.m. we also included a small amount of **protein**, such as an egg or cheese slice or ½ cup of yoghurt, and **fat,** such as a teaspoon of polyunsaturated margarine on our toast, the various food groups noted below could sustain our appetite until midday.

This is not to say that we still wouldn't want a mid-morning snack, especially if we are active or (like children) were growing. However, by eating in this way we are less likely to be eating due to craving sugar.

Figure 3: The effects of digestion rates of foods on blood sugar levels

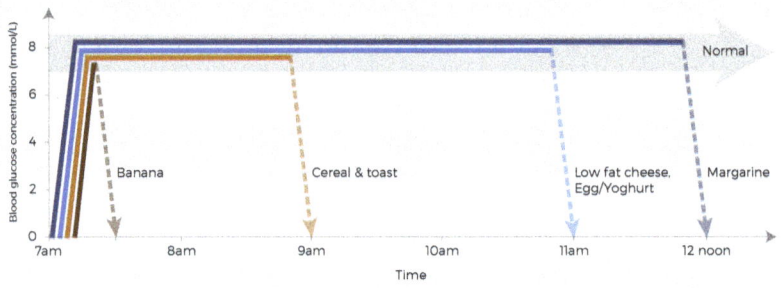

Ref: Stening LB. Nutrition manual for developing rowers. Willson Scott Publishing New Zealand 2005

Ideally, a similar pattern could occur at other meals. For instance, at lunchtime, **carbohydrates** may be eaten in the form of bread, fruit, or salad; **protein** may be contributed by a portion of fish, cheese, egg, or chicken; and the **fat** contributed by such foods as margarine, nuts, or seeds.

At dinner, **carbohydrate** might be eaten as a potato, rice, pasta, or vegetables and fruit. **Protein** could be contributed by meat, poultry, fish, eggs, or beans. Some **fat** could be included from oil in cooking, marinades, or salad dressing, etc.

Generally, extra protein is not required as an in-between snack. However, carbohydrate in the form of fruit or a sandwich or small muffin with a milk drink can supply extra energy, particularly if children are involved in sporting activities.

The Glycaemic Index

The Glycaemic Index (GI) ranks carbohydrate-rich foods as high, medium, or low according to their actual effect on blood glucose (i.e. blood sugar) levels. This index ranks foods on a scale from 0 to 100.

Foods with a high GI (70–100) release their energy rapidly within ½ to 1 hour after being eaten, while foods with a lower GI (< 50) tend to release energy more slowly within a two-hour period, thereby providing more sustainable energy for better health. Food processing appears to raise the GI, which is why eating foods whole is preferrable to the juicing of food.

There are situations before, during and after sporting activities, where the use of high and low GI foods can improve sporting performance. See Time your eating for better performance (bit.ly/2jQ7e8o).

However, on a daily basis, children undergoing normal physical activity (<45–60 minutes) do not need high-GI foods for spurts of energy. In fact, an over-consumption of foods such as sports drinks, lollies, and chips can lead to peaks and troughs in blood sugar that may lead to sugar cravings, a greater risk of dental caries, type 2 diabetes, and obesity.

For good health:

> Enjoy whole foods as much as possible.
> Choose breakfast cereals that contain barley, oats (e.g. porridge), wheat

or rice bran.
- Choose grainy breads containing whole seeds, barley, or oats rather than white or brown bread.
- Include legumes and pulses (e.g. beans, lentils and peas).
- Eat foods that are high in fibre, as these slow the digestion and absorption of carbohydrates, particularly when also combined with protein-rich foods.

Further reading

- For a list of the GI content of foods, refer to the University of Sydney Glycemic Index website (bit.ly/2jpuUVh)
- Time your eating for better performance (bit.ly/2jQ7e8o)

Ten ways to stay healthy

Now that you understand about energy and why it is so important not to miss meals, these ten tips can help to improve the quality of your family's food intake.

1. Eat breakfast to kick-start your day

- Choose a breakfast cereal that contains less than 15gm sugar/100g, such as Weetbix™, porridge, or bran cereal.
- Avoid sprinkling sugar on top of cereals as this obviously bumps up the total sugar load unnecesaryily.
- Add some fruit and yoghurt, or a slice of toast with either cheese or an egg on top.
- Choose a wholegrain bread with additional fibre that will keep you feeling full for longer.
- When children are growing, breakfast makes up ⅓ of their daily food intake, so it is very important. Even if they sleep in at the weekends and don't make breakfast until after 10 a.m., just shift lunch nearer to 1 or 2 p.m. Otherwise, they will be snacking all afternoon.
- If your child regularly skips breakfast, think about the reasons why this happens. Maybe they need to arrange breakfast items the night before, or take a cheese or egg sandwich to school for morning interval instead.

2. Eat more bread and cereals

Grains are an important source of energy that provide dietary fibre for bowel health and some B group vitamins for building healthy nerves, skin, and the immune system.

Many of these nutrients are lost when grains are highly processed, so choose whole grain versions where possible as these will also be more filling.

When milk is added to cereals, they absorb moisture and swell. As they are eaten and pass through the gut they are digested — but not completely. Some cereals contribute more digestion-resistant and fermentation-resistant remnants, to survive passage through the gut, than other cereals. The amount that survives passage, and the amount of water it binds, contributes to "faecal bulking".

Cereals that bulk up the most help us control body weight, as they make us feel more full. Bulky cereals also soften stools, preventing constipation and bowel cancer, aid the growth of beneficial bacteria in the gut, and help to lower cholesterol.

Note

- Since this research was undertaken, some of these cereals have been reformulated to include oat and wheat bran for added fibre, as you will read on the food label.
- While a small amount of bran can make a healthy contribution to a diet, more is not better. Bran cereals are very bulky and contain a substance called **phytate** which can reduce the absorption of calcium, iron, and zinc. So only ½ cup is recommended each day for adults and children 5 years and over and (as with all cereals) it needs to be accompanied by a good intake of fluids throughout the day.
- Parents of children who are wheat intolerant and following gluten-free diets can enrich their childs dietary fibre intake by adding rice bran to their cereals each day.

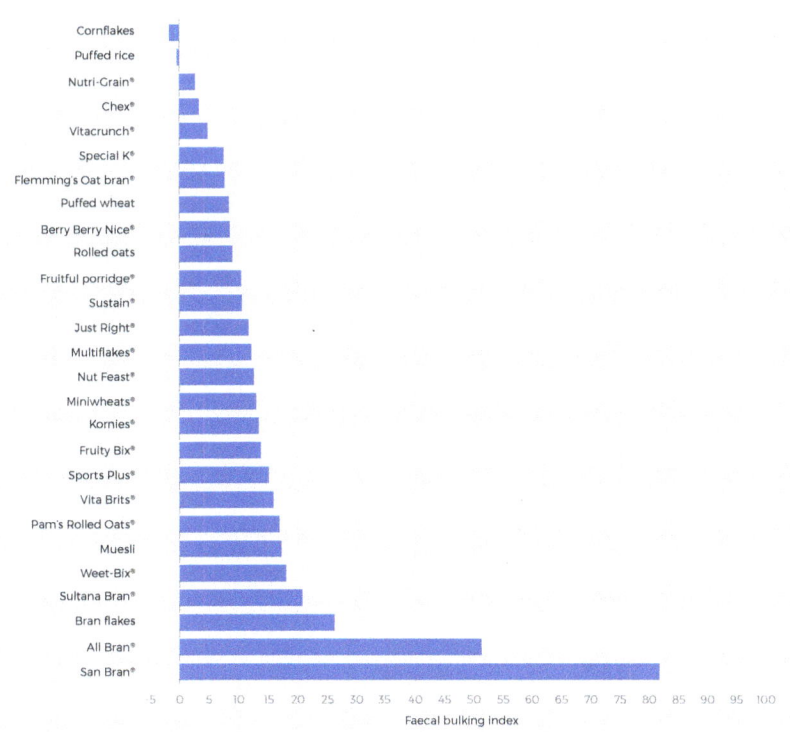

Figure 4: The faecal bulking effect of Australasian breakfast cereals

Ref: Monro J. Faecal Bulking of Australasian Cereals Asian Pacific Journal of Clinical Nutrition 2002 11 (3):176–185

For more information, refer to:

> Boosting your fibre intake offers huge health benefits (bit.ly/2jprGRn)
> Is going gluten free a healthy food choice? (bit.ly/2jOCyqA)
> Feeling full is the secret to weight loss (bit.ly/2kMFR39)

3. Enjoy fruits and vegetables

> Raw fruits and vegetables are good sources of Vitamin C and dietary fibre.
> Brightly coloured fruits and vegetables are full of antioxidant nutrients which protect our immune system.
> Yellow, orange, and red vegetables contain beta-carotene which forms Vitamin A and aids healthy skin, eyes, and the immune system. To increase your intake, it can really help to include a few cherry tomatoes or carrot sticks into your lunch, along with a serving of pumpkin, carrots, capsicum, tomato, or kumara into your evening meals.
> Green leafy vegetables are an important source of iron and folate that improve memory and mood. It can really improve your wellbeing to add lettuce to sandwiches and wraps, and include spinach in salads, soups, pizzas, and mince dishes.

Further reading

> "Free foods" for hungry children (bit.ly/2kK0nOI)
> Get into fruit and vegetables for optimal health (bit.ly/2kbx4F0)

4. Eat lean meat, chicken, seafood, eggs, legumes, nuts, and seeds

> These foods are an important source of protein for growth.
> They also contribute iron, which attaches to red blood cells and carries oxygen to body cells. Iron is very important for fighting fatigue and aids discrimination and concept learning.
> Limit the use of processed meats, luncheon, salami, bacon, and ham as these contain high levels of salt, saturated fat, and preservatives; over time, these may increase the risk of heart disease and some forms of cancer.
> Legumes also contain protein, and can be included into the diet as cooked dried beans, peas, and lentils.

> Vegetarians need a wide range of breads and cereals, fruits and vegetables, legumes (peas, beans, and lentils) milk, eggs, nuts, and seeds. If your child does not drink cow's milk then use soy or rice milk enriched with calcium and vitamin B12.
> Vegan diets can limit children's intake of energy, protein, and key vitamins and minerals essential for growth and development. As nutrient requirements vary according to children's age and activity levels, do talk with your doctor or dietitian before undertaking dietary supplementation.

Further reading
> Iron makes us happy are you getting enough? (bit.ly/2kJYEsR)
> Vegetarians face extra hurdles (bit.ly/2klSbH4)

5. Reduce your intake of trans and saturated fats

There is much publicity in linking fat (particularly trans and saturated fat) with heart disease, stroke, and some forms of cancer. This has led many people to believe that **all** fat is bad. This is not so.

In the correct amounts some fats are essential for good health. They provide energy, insulate our body, coat our brain and nerve tissue, carry and help the absorption of fat-soluble vitamins (A, D, E, and K), and help to build the structure of cell walls.

Fats also add flavor and a moist texture to foods. Since fats digest slowly, they provide a feeling of fullness.

In simple terms, there are basically three main types of fats in our diet: saturated fats, trans fats, and unsaturated fats.

Saturated fats

These large droplets of fat are solid at room temperature. They encourage the body to make the bad LDL cholesterol which, over time, can collect on the lining of our arteries, causing them to narrow and restrict blood flow. This action increases blood pressure and raises blood cholesterol levels, while also increasing the risk of heart disease, obesity, and some forms of cancer.

While cardiovascular disease is rarely seen in children, the disease process (e.g. atherosclerosis or narrowing of the arteries) begins in childhood. Diets high in saturated fat have also been found to impair learning acquisition and memory.

Saturated fats are mostly found in fried foods, in the white fat on meat and chicken skin and full fat dairy products (single or double cream, butter, whole milk, and cheese). Coconut oil, coconut cream, and lard are also high in saturated fat.

Trans fats

Trans fats are created when vegetables oils are hardened by hydrogenation. This process is designed to extend the shelf life of food products. Trans fats are often used as a cheaper alternative to butter in cakes, biscuits, and pastries, and for deep frying.

Trans fats can also be found naturally in small amounts in meat and dairy products such as full cream milk and butter.

The main concern is that not only do trans fats raise the bad LDL cholesterol, they also lower the good HDL cholesterol, thereby increasing the risk of heart disease.

Unsaturated fats

Unsaturated fats (e.g. polyunsaturated and monounsaturated) are smaller droplets of fat that are liquid at room temperature, and that travel through the blood system more easily. These reduce the risk of heart disease and at a mental level, they aid cognition and reduce depression.

Some fats such as alpha-linolenic fatty acids (omega 3) and linoleic (omega 6) cannot be synthesised by the body and so need to be provided by the diet.

Vegetarians need adequate levels of these fatty acids which act as precursors for long-chain fatty acids found in animal foods. Good sources of alpha linolenic and linoleic acid can be found in plant-based spreads such as nuts and seeds (chia, flax/linseed, soybean).

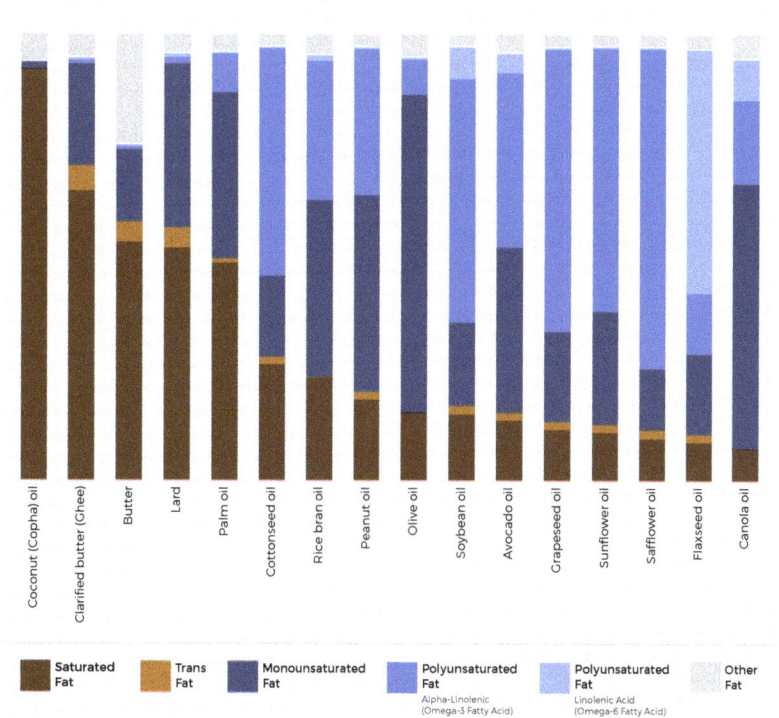

Figure 5: The composition of different types of fat

Ref: Foodworks 2015

Good sources of long-chain omega 3 fatty acids can be found in oily fish (salmon, tuna, sardines, Kahawai, mackerel, and herrings), as well as in unsalted raw or dry roasted nuts, seeds, and plant oils.

How to achieve a healthier balance of fats in the diet

For good health, it is important to not only reduce the intake of saturated and trans fat but also to increase the proportion of poly and monounsaturated fats in the diet while keeping the level of total fat in the diet to around 25 to 30% of daily energy intake.

> Choose lean meat (beef, lamb, pork or venison) and poultry, and trim the visible fat before cooking and eating. Also try to grill meats rather than frying them.
> Eggs can be eaten daily but it is healthier to scramble, boil, or poach these rather than fry eggs.
> For children who are two years or older and growing well, choose reduced or low-fat milks such as those colour-coded in light blue (1.5% fat), yellow (0.1% fat) or green (0.3% fat), and low-fat milk products such as yoghurt, Edam, cottage, or ricotta cheese.
> Use less fat in cooking and replace butter and lard with oils such as sunflower, canola, and olive oil.
> When choosing spreads, read food labels to ensure that the margarine you are buying contains poly or monounsaturated fats.
> In Australia and New Zealand, look out for foods with the Heart Foundation tick mark. Over 25 varieties of margarines have been approved because they have <1% trans fats and <28% saturated fat content. Butter, in comparison, has 4% trans fats and 50% saturated fat content.
> Other spreads such as hummus, tahini, avocado, and nut butters are lower in saturated fat and higher in polyunsaturated fat than butter, although not quite as high in polyunsaturated fat as can be found in polyunsaturated margarines. If using nut butters, choose varieties low in salt and sugar and limit intake to serving size/age (see "Table 3: The

daily allowance of healthy fats required by children of different age groups").
> If adults in the family are using plant sterol spreads, check with your doctor before giving these to children.

Overall, choose fats with the most poly and monounsaturated fats and the lowest levels of trans and saturated fats.

Further reading
> How to increase the good fats in your diet (bit.ly/2kOIqOa)
> Can coconut improve our health? (bit.ly/2jpsFkx)

6. Eat takeaways less than once a week

Takeaways are foods not prepared at home, including bakery lunch items such as pies, savouries, and slices. These foods invariably have high levels of saturated fat, salt, and sugar; however, the following tips may help to reduce the load for the odd times that you do eat them:

> If buying a takeaway for dinner, keep to regular serving sizes rather than up-sizing the meal.
> If buying chips, choose wedges, as these have less surface area on which to trap fat than shoestring chips or crinkle-cut versions.
> Instead of fish and chips, order a hamburger and extend this meal with beetroot, pineapple, coleslaw, or salad. Avoid the impulse to layer on more fat in the form of extra cheese, egg, or meat.
> Low-fat alternatives include options such as Subway ˚ sandwiches; enchiladas; wraps; thin-crust vegetarian pizzas; Asian-style meals with boiled (rather than fried) rice and vegetables; a baked potato with meat plus beans and salad; souvlaki or sushi.

Further reading
> Healthy ideas for family takeaway meals (bit.ly/2kONG4j)

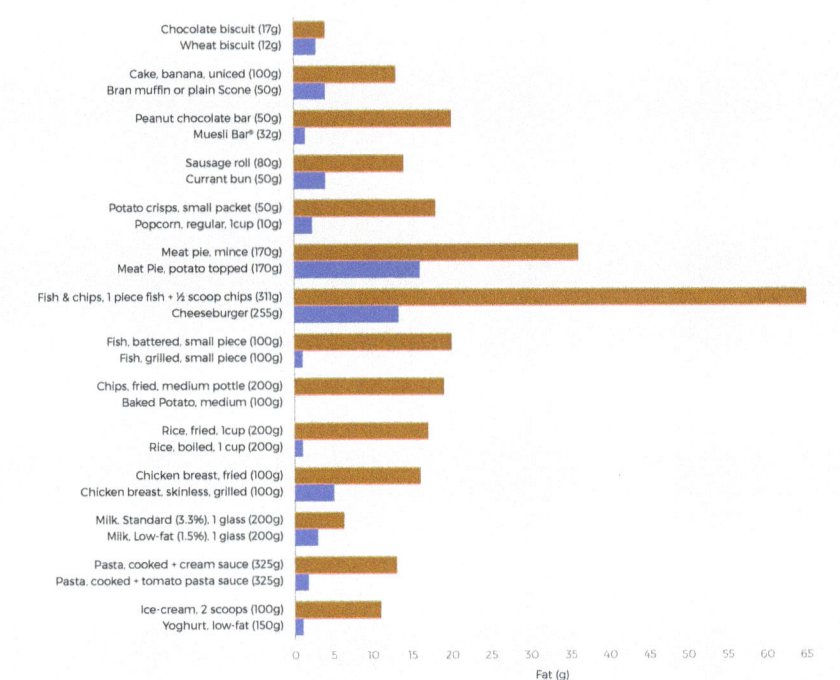

Figure 6: The fat content of average servings of various takeaway meals and snacks

Ref: Foodworks 2015

7. Make snacks healthy

Growing children often need to eat in-between meals, particularly if they are very active or playing sport. Healthy snacks might include:

> Yoghurt
> Fresh fruit
> Vegetable sticks with hummus

- A low-fat cheese or Vegemite®/Marmite® sandwich
- Small fruit scones or muffins (using banana, carrot, or berries to flavour rather than chocolate, coconut or cheese varieties)
- Unsalted nuts (1 to 2 Tbsp)
- Muesli bars (Note: these can pack a high dose of calories and sugar, so are best chosen with care and according to their use such as a snack for sport or an endurance event). See "Further reading" below.
- A fruit smoothie made with low-fat milk, vanilla, berries, or ½ banana can make a good mid-afternoon or after sport snack, but avoid adding ice cream, yoghurt, or protein powders as these unnecessarily increase the protein, sodium, and sugar load.

How to reduce the sugar content of snack foods

Snack foods can be a major source of sugar in the diet contributing to the risk of obesity, Type 2 diabetes, and poor dental health. So how much sugar should we be eating?

The New Zealand Ministry of Health recommends that we consume between 45 to 65% of our daily energy from carbohydrate (starches and sugars) but that for good health we should limit the intake of free sugars (also known as *extrinsic* or *added* sugars) to less than 10% of total energy intake.

In 2015, the World Health Organisation (WHO) recommended a greater reduction of free sugars to no more than 5% of free sugars per day (6 tsp).

Free sugars are defined as mono and disaccharides that are added to food by manufacturers, cooks, and consumers plus sugars naturally present in foods such as honey, syrups, and fruit juices.

Most of our carbohydrates should therefore come from *intrinsic* sugars that are bound to the cell walls of whole grain breads and cereals, fruits (two pieces per day), vegetables, and legumes. These sugars, along with the milk sugar lactose (in unflavoured milks), are considered healthy because their absorption tends to be slower and they are accompanied by other essential nutrients.

For better health, the Australian Dietary Guidelines also recommend reducing the intake of discretionary foods of limited nutritional value, such as cakes, biscuits (sweet and savoury), potato chips and crisps, corn chips, rice crackers, chocolate, confectionery (candy), and sugar-sweetened soft drinks and fruit juice (irrespective of their added sugar content).

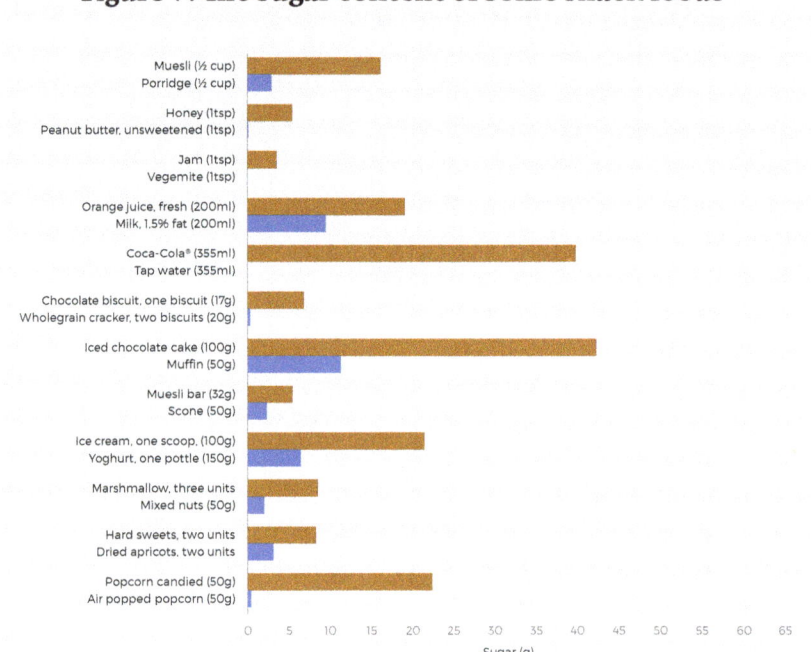

Figure 7: The sugar content of some snack foods

Ref: Foodworks 2015

Parents of children who are overweight or obese should note that some foods considered to be healthy, such as muesli bars, muesli, and nuts, can be very high in energy; irrespective of their sugar or fat content, these should be limited until a healthier weight is achieved.

Sugar and dental health

When foods or drinks containing sugars are eaten, these molecules combine with saliva and the bacteria in the mouth and lead to a build-up of plaque on teeth, which can lead in turn to demineralization of tooth enamel and dental caries.

An excess of sugar can also lead to gum disease which, if left untreated, can develop into periodontitis, a serious gum infection that damages the soft tissue and destroys the bone supporting teeth. Once in the blood, the bacteria associated with periodontitis can travel through the body invading joints, soft tissues, and vital organs such as the heart, liver, and kidneys.

Dental health is a serious matter. Disease is easily preventable when parents encourage their children to consume foods and drinks with fewer added sugars, to drink water after meals or snacks, and to brush their teeth as soon as possible after eating main meals using a pea-sized amount of fluoride toothpaste and water.

Further reading

- › Sugar control is essential for better health (bit.ly/2jpu9v8)
- › What's the fuss about fructose (bit.ly/2klVZZb)
- › Muesli and sports bars can aid performance (bit.ly/2jpjmky)
- › Are you a sneaky snacker? (bit.ly/2jQ1snd)
- › Athletes protect your winning smile (bit.ly/2kOZdAC)

8. Drink plenty of fluids

Water

Water is vital to life, contributing 50 to 60% of our body weight. Just a 1% to 2% drop in hydration can reduce physical performance by 20%, yet we can dream up any excuse to avoid drinking it.

For instance, people will say, "I can't be bothered", "It makes me want to go to the toilet", or "I forgot." The bottom line is that if you drink enough total fluid each day you will feel more alert and full of energy:

> - Fluids deliver energy around your body while collecting and removing waste products. So if you don't drink water, you will feel tired and sluggish and gain unnecessary weight.
> - Fluids help to balance the electrolytes in our body that regulate blood pressure; they also assist temperature regulation and aid the chemical reactions that govern digestion, absorption, and excretion.
> - Water is cheap and easily accessible; water and milk are the fluids of choice for growing children.

Milk and milk products (cheese and yoghurt)

> - Milk contains protein, B-group vitamins, and calcium, all of which are important for growth and bone health.
> - Drinking milk after exercise assists rehydration and body repair.
> - Serve milk after meals or as a healthy in-between meal snack.
> - Choose low-fat milk, as it contains more protein and calcium than standard milk while offering fewer calories/kilojoules.
> - Encourage children to enjoy the natural flavour of milk rather than adding sugar or flavouring.
> - If children are unable to tolerate dairy products then choose soy, rice, almond, goat's or ewe's milk enriched with calcium and Vitamin B12.

Fruit juice

Fruit juice is not recommended because it is acidic and contains high amounts of sugar (natural and added), factors that may contribute to dental caries. If drinking juice, dilute it to ½ water and ½ juice, and take it with a meal rather than as a between-meal snack.

Carbonated drinks

Carbonated drinks are high in sugar, energy (calories), and may contain caffeine. These should be only taken occasionally (i.e. less than once per week).

Sports drinks

Sports drinks are not required for children's normal sporting activity. Prior to puberty, fluid losses are usually small, and milk and water are sufficient. However, adolescents taking part in vigorous senior sporting endeavours lasting more than two hours may require an extra carbohydrate infusion. A sports dietitian can help you ensure that the carbohydrates in these drinks are taken as part of an overall sports programme.

Energy drinks

Energy drinks and shots are not recommended for children. These can contain high levels of sugar, amino acids, electrolytes, herbal extracts such as ginseng and guarana, and unnecessary caffeine stimulants which can lead to insomnia and mood swings.

Alcohol

Alcohol is not recommended. If you choose to drink, drink only a little; eat some food, don't binge drink, and do not drive.

Note

Milk and water are the preferred drinks for children. For guidelines on quantities for various age groups refer to "Table 2: The number of servings of food groups required by children of different age groups."

Further reading

> What are our children drinking? (bit.ly/2klLd50)
> What's to drink? (bit.ly/2kK4pqy)
> Drink milk for better health (bit.ly/2klMKId)
> Milk matters (bit.ly/2kJZHsB)

9. Sleep 10 to 12 hours per day

Getting plenty of sleep helps with learning, weight management, and feeling happy. Lost sleep puts all of us at a greater risk of weight gain. This is because there is an increase in the hormone *ghrelin* (that makes us hungry) and a decrease in the hormone *leptin* (that makes us feel full).

Sleep also aids the growth rate in children because it allows energy to be diverted away from physical activity, and redirects it to growth and development.

Try these tips to improve the quality of your family's sleep:

> Set a regular bedtime routine.
> Remove from the bedroom things that might cause distractions to sleep such as electronics (including any television, computers, game consoles, or cellphones).
> Limit screen time to less than two hours per day; encourage more physical activity, as this can improve the quality of sleep.
> Research has found that caffeine can increase the time it takes to get to sleep and also to reduce the total sleep time. Children are more sensitive to caffeine than adults because of their smaller body size which can make them more susceptible to its stimulatory effect. So pay attention to possible sources of caffeine in your child's diet such as energy drinks, tea, and coffee consumption.

Further reading

> Do your kids a favour — turn off the TV (bit.ly/2jpvfqW)

10. Keep active

Keeping children active aids growth and development by strengthening bones and muscles, not to mention hand-eye co-ordination and balance. Staying active also helps children to develop social skills and self-confidence.

Most parents assume that children get enough physical activity at school and whilst playing. However, research shows that children are becoming more sedentary. Here are some tips to help:

> Aim for 60 minutes of exercise each day — the more vigorous the better.
> Increase incidental exercise each day by taking the stairs and avoiding the elevator; park further from shops and school so the family can walk more.
> Encourage children to join a club activity such as karate, basketball, badminton, softball, or soccer.
> Try to make family activities more fun by walking, tramping, or playing ball sports together at the weekend or during holidays.
> If sharing celebrations such as birthdays or barbecues, plan the mealtime around a group activity such as swimming, bowling, ice skating, cricket, or basketball to keep everyone moving.
> If children have spare time over the weekend or holidays, they could help out with jobs and activities at home: mow the lawns, plant a vegetable garden, maybe help you stack some wood.
> They could also go for a run, swim, walk, or bike ride with a friend.
> If children become serious about a sport, practising for more than 3 to 4 hours per week after school, they should contact us or a sports dietitian to learn about eating before, during, and post-recovery exercise.

Further reading

> Playtime helps combat childhood obestity (bit.ly/2jQ0Jmi)
> Tips to move you off the couch (bit.ly/2klUfOS)

Healthy baseline meal plan

Sample plan for school children

Breakfast

Cereal with low-fat milk
Small piece of fruit
Boiled egg or cheese slice or pottle of yoghurt
1 slice medium wholegrain toast with thin spread of margarine and peanut butter or Vegemite*
Drink of milk or water

Mid-morning

Small scone or muffin
Milk or water

Lunch

Pita bread or sandwiches with salad and tuna, chicken, or cheese etc.
Vegetable sticks and hummus
Piece of raw fruit
Water

Mid-afternoon

Crackers or fruit loaf
Low-fat milkshake

Dinner

Small serving of meat, fish, chicken, or vegetarian option
Potato, rice, or pasta
Tossed green salad or vegetables
Yoghurt and fruit (optional)
Water

Supper

Hot milk drink

Quantities

The quantities offered depend on the age of the child (Refer to "Table 2: The number of servings of food groups required by children of different age groups"). Also, cultural differences may alter the types of foods chosen. For instance, boiled rice may be preferred to breakfast cereal or toast for Asian or Indian families, though a source of protein should still be added.

For guidance with specific food quantities and meal plans tailored to meet the needs of your child, contact us (bit.ly/2klI4Sy) or your local paediatric dietitian.

Allergies and intolerances

Even if your child has been medically diagnosed with a food allergy or intolerance, e.g. gluten or lactose intolerance, this pattern of eating need not change. Simply use gluten-free products when baking and lactose-free milk.

Avoid self-diagnosing your child's conditions as this can lead to shortfalls in important nutrients, which may hamper your child's growth or possibly leave undiagnosed a greater health problem.

Talk to your doctor and contact us or your local dietitian for practical help, meal, and recipe ideas.

Hard snack foods warning

Do not give hard snack foods such as whole nuts or large seeds until children are at least 5 years old, to reduce the risk of choking.

Dietary supplements

Children should not be given any dietary supplements unless on the recommendation of their doctor.

Older children taking part in sporting endeavours should also be aware of the regulations regarding dietary supplements and sport.

Further reading

> - Sports supplements should be taken with care (bit.ly/2kK2OAQ)
> - Food and Nutrition Guidelines for Healthy Children and Young People (Aged 2-18 years): A background paper (bit.ly/2kbyIGG)
> - Australian Dietary Guidelines (bit.ly/2km7ZJp)

What does one serving mean?

Serving sizes will vary according to the type of food considered. Notice how fruit and vegetables carry a lot fewer kilojoules than the other food groups; they are also bulkier and very filling.

Vegetables

A standard serving is around 75g (100-350kJ):

> - ½ cup cooked green or orange vegetables (e.g. broccoli, spinach, carrot, or pumpkin)

Table 2: The number of servings of food groups required by children of different age groups

Age	Vegetables and legumes/beans	Fruit	Grain (cereal)	Lean meat, poultry, fish, eggs, nuts and seeds, and legumes/beans	Milk and milk products
Toddlers					
1-2 years	2-3	½	4	1	1-1½
Boys					
2-3 years	2½	1	4	1	1½
4-8 years	4½	1½	4	1½	2
9-11 years	5	2	5	2½	2½
12-13 years	5½	2	6	2½	3½
14-18 years	5½	2	7	2½	3½
Girls					
2-3 years	2½	1	4	1	1½
4-8 years	4½	1½	4	1½	1½
9-11 years	5	2	4	2½	3
12-13 years	5	2	5	2½	3½
14-18 years	5	2	7	2½	3½

* Nut pastes are recommended instead of whole nuts and seeds because of the potential choking risk

- ½ cup cooked dried or canned beans, peas, or lentils
- 1 cup leafy or raw salad vegetables
- ½ cup sweetcorn
- ½ medium potato or starchy vegetable (e.g. sweet potato, taro, or cassava)
- 1 medium tomato

Fruit

A standard serving is around 150g (350kJ):

> 1 medium apple, banana, orange, or pear
> 2 small apricots, kiwifruits, or plums
> 1 cup diced or canned fruit (no added sugar) or only occasionally
> 125ml (½ cup) fruit juice (no added sugar)
> 30g dried fruit (e.g. 4 dried apricot halves, 1½ tablespoons of sultanas)

Grains

A standard serving is (500kJ):

> 1 slice (40g) bread
> ½ medium (40g) roll or flat bread
> ½ cup (75-120g) cooked rice, pasta, noodles, barley, buckwheat, semolina, polenta, bulgar, or quinoa.
> ½ cup (120g) cooked porridge
> ⅔ cup (30g) wheat cereal flakes
> ½ cup (30g) muesli
> 3 (35g) crispbreads
> 1 (60g) crumpet
> 1 small (35g) English muffin or scone

Choose grains or cereal foods, mostly whole grain and/or high cereal fibre varieties.

Lean meat and poultry, fish, eggs, nuts and seeds, and legumes/beans

A standard serving (500–600kJ) looks like this:

> 65g cooked lean red meats, e.g. beef, lamb, veal, pork, goat, or kangaroo (around 90-100g raw)

- 80g cooked lean poultry, e.g. chicken or turkey (around 100g raw)
- 100g cooked fish fillet (around 115g raw) or one small can of fish
- 2 large (120g) eggs
- 1 cup (150g) cooked or canned legumes/beans, e.g. lentils, chickpeas, or split peas
- 170g tofu
- 30g nuts, seeds, peanut or almond butter, tahini, or other nut or seed paste (no added salt). This amount for nuts and seeds gives approximately the same amount of energy as the other foods in this group but will provide less protein, iron, or zinc.*

* Only to be used occasionally as a substitute for other foods in the group

Milk, cheese, yoghurt, cheese and/or alternatives

A standard serving (500-600kJ):

- 1 cup (250ml) fresh, UHT long life, reconstituted powered milk or buttermilk
- ½ cup (120ml) evaporated milk
- 2 slices (40g) or 4×3×2 cm cube (40g) of hard cheese, such as cheddar or Edam
- ½ cup ricotta cheese
- ¾ cup (200g) yoghurt
- 1 cup (250ml) soy, rice, or other cereal drink with at least 100mg of added calcium per 100ml

Choose mostly reduced fat varieties. If you do not eat any food from this group, try the following foods which contain around the same amount of calcium as a serving of milk, yoghurt, cheese, or alternatives. (Note: the kilojoule content of some of these servings - especially nuts - is higher, so watch this if trying to lose weight.)

- 100g almonds with skin

> 60g sardines, canned in water
> ½ cup (100g) canned pink salmon with bones
> 100g firm tofu (check the label as calcium levels vary)

Healthy fats

A daily allowance for additional unsaturated fats from spreads, oils, nuts or seeds is also recommended to aid the development of brain and nerve tissue.

Table 3: The daily allowance of healthy fats required by children of different age groups

Age	Daily allowance for additional unsaturated fats
1–2 years	7–10g
2–3 years	4.5g
4–11 years	7–10g
12–13 years	11–15g
14–18 years	14–20g

* Nut pastes are recommended instead of whole nuts and seeds because of the potential choking risk

Fluid Requirements

These are minimum levels for age. Please note that fluid requirements will vary acording to factors such as the climate, altitude, and health and activity levels of the child.

Table 4: The daily allowance of fluids required by children of different age groups

Age	Males' daily fluid allowance	Females' daily fluid allowance
2-3 years	1.0 litres	1.0 litres
4-8 years	1.2 litres	1.2 litres
9-13 years	1.6 litres	1.4 litres
14-18 years	1.9 litres	1.6 litres

Milk and water are the preferrable drinks for children. See the guidelines for milk intake above under "Milk, cheese, yoghurt, cheese and/or alternatives".

References

> Food and Nutrition Guidelines for Healthy Children and Young People (Aged 2-18 years): A background paper (bit.ly/2kbyIGG)
> Australian food guidelines (bit.ly/2kOXiMN)

Shopping tips

Good nutrition begins in the supermarket trolley. Understanding which foods make the healthiest use of your food dollars today will also benefit your family's long-term health and wealth.

> - Make a list and try to stick to it.
> - Eat before you leave home to reduce distraction by the impulse buys of confectionery items, which are strategically placed by the checkout to tempt shoppers as they leave.
> - Avoid shopping at peak times when there are more people and distractions, which may make you buy more or buy less healthy grocery items. If this is difficult because of work commitments, then consider online shopping where you can be more specific about the quantities of foods needed.
> - Be aware of the advertising, promotions, discounts, and food samples that are all designed to sell you more of what you do not need.
> - Only buy 'specials' that you need and can consume at your normal rate. For example, buying a two-week supply of oranges because they are on 'special' will not save you money if you consume them all in one week.
> - Be aware that food producers pay more for eye-level shelving in supermarkets. This cost is added to the price of any food or drink product.
> - Be a conservationist — remember to take your shopping bags with you to minimize the use of plastic carrier bags.

Reading food labels

The information on food labels will vary from one country to another. New Zealand and Australia have joined forces under the Australia New Zealand Food Standard Code (ANZFSA) to develop standards covering nutrition, health and related claims. See "Further reading" for label reading information in the UK, USA and China.

Information on food labels

The Nutrition Information Panel (NIP)

This panel must show the serving size and number of servings in the packet. It should also clearly display the nutritional content per serving and per 100g (or 100ml if liquid) for energy (kilojoules/kilocalories), protein, fat, saturated fat, carbohydrate, sugars and sodium (the salt component in the product).

The exception to a NIP is if the packets are too small to display a NIP (e.g. chewing gum), if foods have very low significance to nutrient value such as a herb or spice, or if the food is made at the point of sale such as a bakery.

Table 5: Nutrition information panel

NUTRITION INFORMATION (Average)
Serving Size: 50g (approx ½ cup)
Servings per pack: 12

	Quantity per serving	Quantity per 100g
Energy (kJ)	780	1560
(Cal)	187	373
Protein (g)	5.2	10.3
Fat, Total (g)	3.5	6.9
— Saturated fat (g)	0.9	1.8
Carbohydrate, Total (g)	31.1	62.2
— Sugars (g)	10.5	21
Dietary Fibre (g)	4	9.1
Sodium (mg)	28	55
Potassium (mg)	230	460
Iron (mg)	1.79 (14%)*	3.4
Magnesium (mg)	53 (16%)*	105

* Percentage of Recommended Dietary Intake (RDI)
Ingredients: Cereals (63%), Wholegrain cereals (57%), oats (42%), wheat, rye, buckwheat, barley flakes, wheat bran, rice flour, fruit (22%), seeds (4%), raisins, milk, soy

Ingredient list

This lists items in order of greatest percentage of content, e.g. 'Cereals 63%'.

Name or description of the food

The food must carry an accurate name and description of the food, e.g. 'Natural Muesli Fruit & Seed'.

Recall information

The address details of the manufacturer should be displayed in case the product needs to be recalled.

Information for allergy sufferers

Some food ingredients (e.g. peanut, egg, shellfish, gluten, etc) can cause allergic reactions in susceptible people, so these ingredients must be declared on the food labels - however small the amount.

Food additives

Additives are listed according to their function, name, or code, e.g. 'thickener (pectin)' or 'thickener (440)'. See "Further reading" to access the food additive code.

Date stamping

Any product with a shelf life of less than two years must have a 'best before' date beyond which the product quality would deteriorate. Foods that deteriotate after a certain time, endangering the user's health, must state a 'use by' date with the exception of baked goods. These must stipulate 'baked on' or 'baked for' if their shelf life is less than seven days.

Legibility requirements

Regulations govern the size of print on labels so that they are easy to read. Also, labels must tell the truth as they are backed up by Fair Trading laws and food laws in New Zealand and Australia.

Directions for use and storage

In order to preserve the quality of foods, storage temperatures and conditions may be included.

Country of origin

This is used to determine if all the product came completely from Australia (e.g. 'Product of Australia') or is a composite of products from other countries labelled 'Made in Australia'. New Zealand only labels country of origin on wine.

A quick guide to reading labels

Per 100g

Only use the 100g column of the label when you want to compare the product in hand with another similiar product. Look for products lowest in energy (if you need to lose weight), fat, sugar and sodium, yet highest in fibre.

Table 6: Definitions and range of food claims

Food claim	Definition
'Low energy'	80kJ/100ml liquid, 170kJ/100g solid
'Reduced/Light/Lite'	Contains at least 25% less energy, cholesterol or saturated fat than reference food
'Diet'	Food or fluid contains at least 40% less energy than reference food
'Low fat'	No more than 1.5g/100ml liquid, 3g/100g solid
'Low saturated/trans fat'	No more than 0.75g/100ml liquid, 1.5g/100g solid
'Low cholesterol'	10mg/100ml liquid, 20mg/100g solid
'Low sodium'	120mg/100ml liquid, 120mg/100g solid
'Low sugar'	No more than 2.5g/100ml liquid, 5g/100g solid
'No added'	No salt, sodium or sugar has been added including honey, malt or fruit juice
'Unsweetened'	No added sugar plus food contains no intense sweeteners e.g. sorbitol, manitol, glycerol, xylitol, isomalt, maltitol syrup or lactitol
'Free'	No detectable levels
'Low gluten'	No more than 20mg gluten per 100g solid
'Gluten free'	Should also not contain oats, oat products or malted cereals products
'Low lactose'	No more than 2g per 100g solid
'Increased levels'	Food must contain at least 25% more than the reference food
Special claims	When a special claim is made about a food e.g. good source of iron or magnesiun the food must contain at least 10% of the RDI for that nutrient
'Good sources of protein'	10g/serving
'Good sources of dietary fibre'	4g/serving or 7g/serving (an excellent source
'Good source vitamin/mineral'	No less than 25% RDI
Reference food	A food of the same type to which it is being compared that has not been modified remodeled or processed. The standard regular food e.g. whole milk
RDI	Recommended Dietary Intake sufficient to meet nutrient requirements of nearly all (97-98%) healthy individuals in a particular life stage or gender group.

Per serving

This column will tell you the nutrient content of one serving which is 50g (approx. ½ cup) of cereal in "Table 5: Nutrition information panel."

Label claims

The words and levels used to define the nutrient and ingredient contents in foods are now heavily regulated. See "Table 6: Definitions and range of food claims."

Further reading

> Food Labels: What do they mean? (Food Standards Australia New Zealand) (bit.ly/2kMGdXR) [PDF]
> Additives Overview (Food Standards Australia New Zealand) (bit.ly/2kOGZze)
> Label Detective 2016 (Healthy Food Guide NZ) (bit.ly/2kK1uxP) [PDF]
> Nutrition Facts: Read the Label (US FDA) (bit.ly/2km9EPo) [PDF]
> Food Labels (UK National Health Service) (bit.ly/2jOCxTG)
> Standard for Nutrition Labelling of Prepackaged Foods (Ministry of Health of the People's Republic of China) (bit.ly/2kmaQlY) [PDF]

Front of pack designations

Countries around the world are developing front-of-pack symbols in an attempt to help customers make healthier decisions as they shop.

New Zealand and Australia have adopted the Heart Foundation Healthy heart ticks and also the five-star ratings explained below.

See "Further reading" list for information regarding the 'Multiple Traffic Light' system used in the UK and some European countries and the 'Facts up Front' program in the USA.

The National Heart Foundation 'Pick the Tick' Program

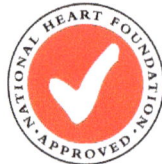 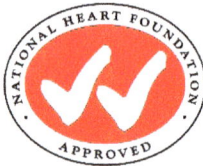

This is a standard to help consumers choose the healthiest food option when buying foods on this type of basis:

> Lower saturated fat, trans fat, salt, energy and (more recently) sugar.
> Ingredients and nutrients that are better for our health, e.g. dietary fibre, calcium, whole grains, and vegetables.

The tick is earned, not bought. The Heart Foundations in New Zealand and Australia have set the standards for different food categories and companies wanting to display this standard on their products submit their food for independent testing. If the product passes the test, then the food company pays the Heart Foundation a license fee to display the tick logo. In this way the scheme is self-funding, and any profits can be directed toward heart research.

The Heart Foundation has now also introduced a double tick to indicate core, whole food items that are good for our health:

> Fruit and vegetables
> Whole grain bread and cereals
> Low and fat-reduced milk and milk products
> Legumes, nuts, seeds, fish and other lean poultry and meat

These foods are regularly reviewed by an independent group of food, nutrition, and health experts and are categorised as a whole food rather than as specific nutrients.

At the time of publication, the National Heart Foundations of Australia and New Zealand have announced that they are phasing out the 'Pick the Tick' program.

The Health Star Rating System

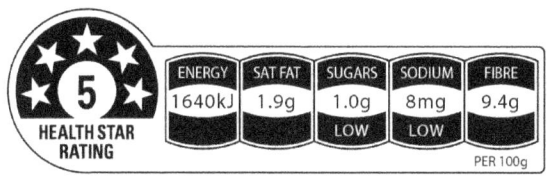

This system is being implemented in New Zealand and Australia and encourages consumers to think about what they are eating or choose a healthier option between packet products of the same category. Foods are rated from ½ to 5 stars per 100g/100ml of product. The greater number of stars, the healthier the food product.

Alongside the star rating, nutrient information is displayed for energy, saturated fat, sugar, sodium, and dietary fibre. Further nutrition information is also available on the Nutrition Information Panel.

Unfortunately it is a voluntary system but over time, it is hoped that more food companies will take part in the scheme. It is important to mention that, even if a food product bears a five-star rating or heart tick, it is still really important to monitor your serving sizes.

Further reading

> - Heart Foundation Tick (National Heart Foundation of New Zealand) (bit.ly/2kOYjnL)
> - How to use Health Star Ratings (Australia/New Zealand) (bit.ly/2kK3arq)
> - Food Labels (UK National Health Service) (bit.ly/2jOCxTG)
> - Facts Up Front Front-of-Pack Labeling Initiative (US Grocery Manufacturers Association) (bit.ly/2jpmJYS)

Food apps

Work is progressing in this field around the world, but in Australia and New Zealand, FoodSwitch is proving popular.

FoodSwitch

This free app was developed by Bupa, The George Institute, and The National Institute for Health Innovation (NIHI). The app is available for both iOS and Android devices and enables consumers to quickly access nutritional information from food labels, as well as to learn about healthier alternative products.

Once opened on a mobile device, a food label barcode can be scanned to produce a clear reading of the food content: energy, fat, saturated fat, sugars, and salt. Within a second, the app will recommend the names of two to five alternative products that are healthier than the one in your hand.

If the product you scan does not appear in the system, the app will prompt you to take photos of the front, rear, and barcode on the pack. This information can then be placed into the FoodSwitch system. In this way the system is constantly kept up-to-date for all users' benefit.

Download

> - FoodSwitch New Zealand (bit.ly/2klNv46)
> - FoodSwitch Australia (bit.ly/2kK5pL6)

Have fun with food

Now that you and your family know the basics of eating food for health and energy, it's important to also have fun with food.

How can we have fun with food?

> Mix things up. Try new varieties of breads, fruits and vegetables.
> Share food ideas with friends, and experiment with different milkshake and breakfast combinations.
> Learn about the food prepared by people of different cultures; be open to trying new recipes and dishes.
> Encourage children to cook a meal at the weekends. It doesn't have to be hard — just a salad or pizza. See if they can develop their own 'signature' dish.
> Teach younger children to count out, measure and weigh fruit and vegetables when shopping and cooking.
> Grow a garden or plant herbs in small pots on the windowsill.
> Teach children to cut vegetables into different shapes and make animals out of raw vegetables using toothpicks to secure its arms, head and legs.

Maintain the fun by staying safe.

> Remind children to wash their hands before handling food and to clean up afterwards.
> Show them how to handle knives with special care, to use pot mit's and oven cloths if handling hot dishes from the oven.
> Always wipe up foods or fluids spilt on the floor to prevent slips and falls.
> Remind your children to check with you before cooking, to ensure that ingredients they want to use are not pre-planned for another meal.

Finally

At the start of this book, I asked you to record your children's food and fluid intake, along with their levels of sleep and exercise. After reviewing this book and the things you need for optimal health and growth, what could they change in order to be a healthier version of themselves?

Remember...
1. They are one of a kind — one body — one mind.
2. No one else is like them.
3. They have heaps of talent, loads of dreams, but only one life.
4. They need to look after it.

Love and best wishes,

Lea

RECIPES

Teaching a child to cook a simple meal or snack is an important way to have fun, build confidence, life skills, and better health.

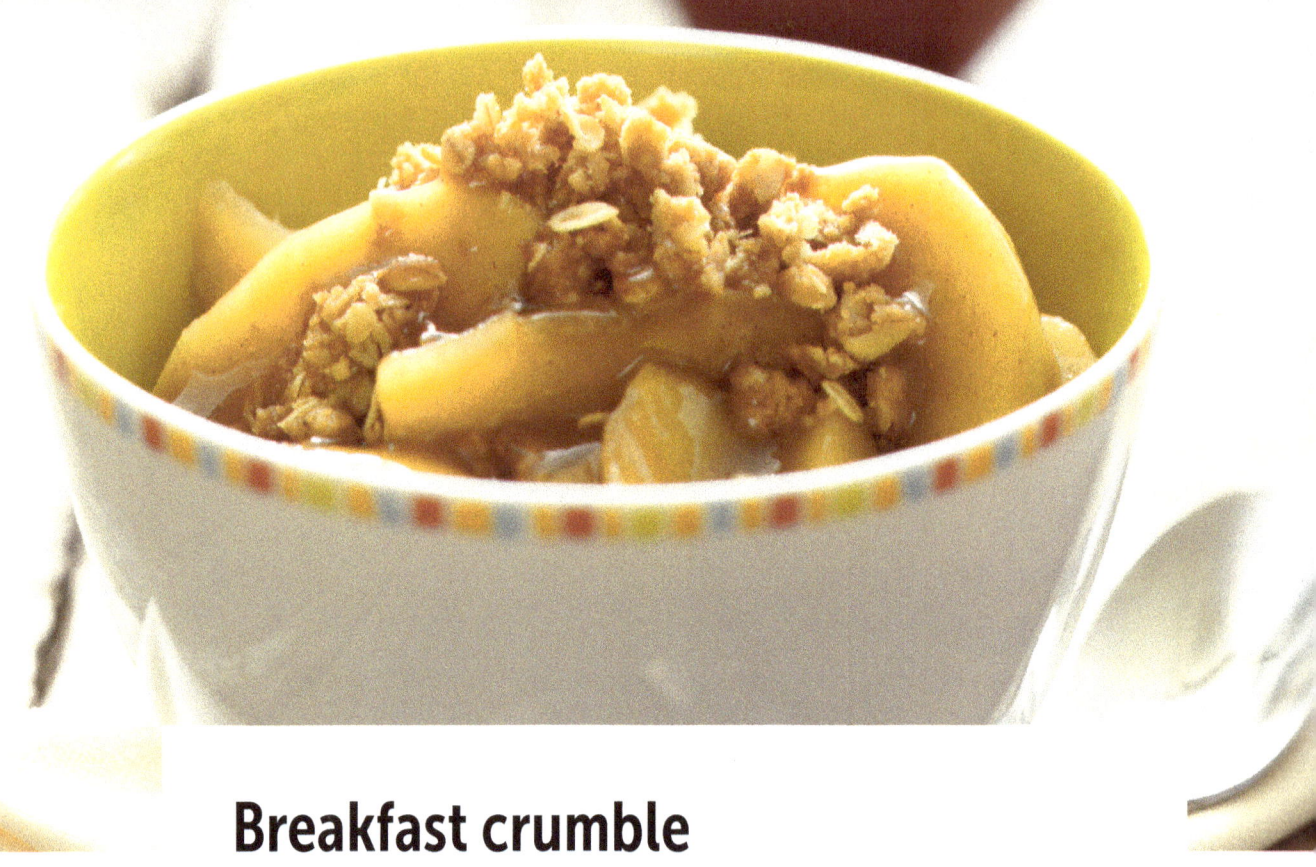

Breakfast crumble

Bran cereals can greatly improve our intake of dietary fibre and B group vitamins important for weight control, bowel health, building immunity, etc. However, finding ways to eat bran can be a challenge at times.

This breakfast is really great! It can be eaten hot or cold and is seriously good with yoghurt. It is also great when using other fruits such as rhubarb, berries, tamarillos, plums, or our 'fruit combo'. Do give it a try; you will never feel hungry mid-morning again.

Ingredients

45g (1½ oz) bran breakfast cereal
1 Tbsp muesli or raw oats
80g (2½ oz) canned or stewed fruit (cooked apple or peaches are good)
⅛ tsp of cinnamon (optional)
125 ml (4 fl oz) low-fat milk
150 ml (5 fl oz) low-fat yoghurt (optional)

Method

1. Place the bran into a bowl; top with fruit, muesli, or oats and the cinnamon.
2. Add the milk.
3. Microwave the bran and fruit for 2 minutes on high.
4. Top with yoghurt and a little more milk if needed.

Serves: 1
Each serving contains: Energy 786kJ/187kcals; Protein 10g; Fat 2.6; Saturated fat 0.6; Carbohydrate 30g; Sodium 308mg

To vary this recipe, in place of the muesli, try some of the new 'ancient grains' oat cereals that combine oats, rye, quinoa, and millet offering more iron and B group vitamins with less salt and sugar.

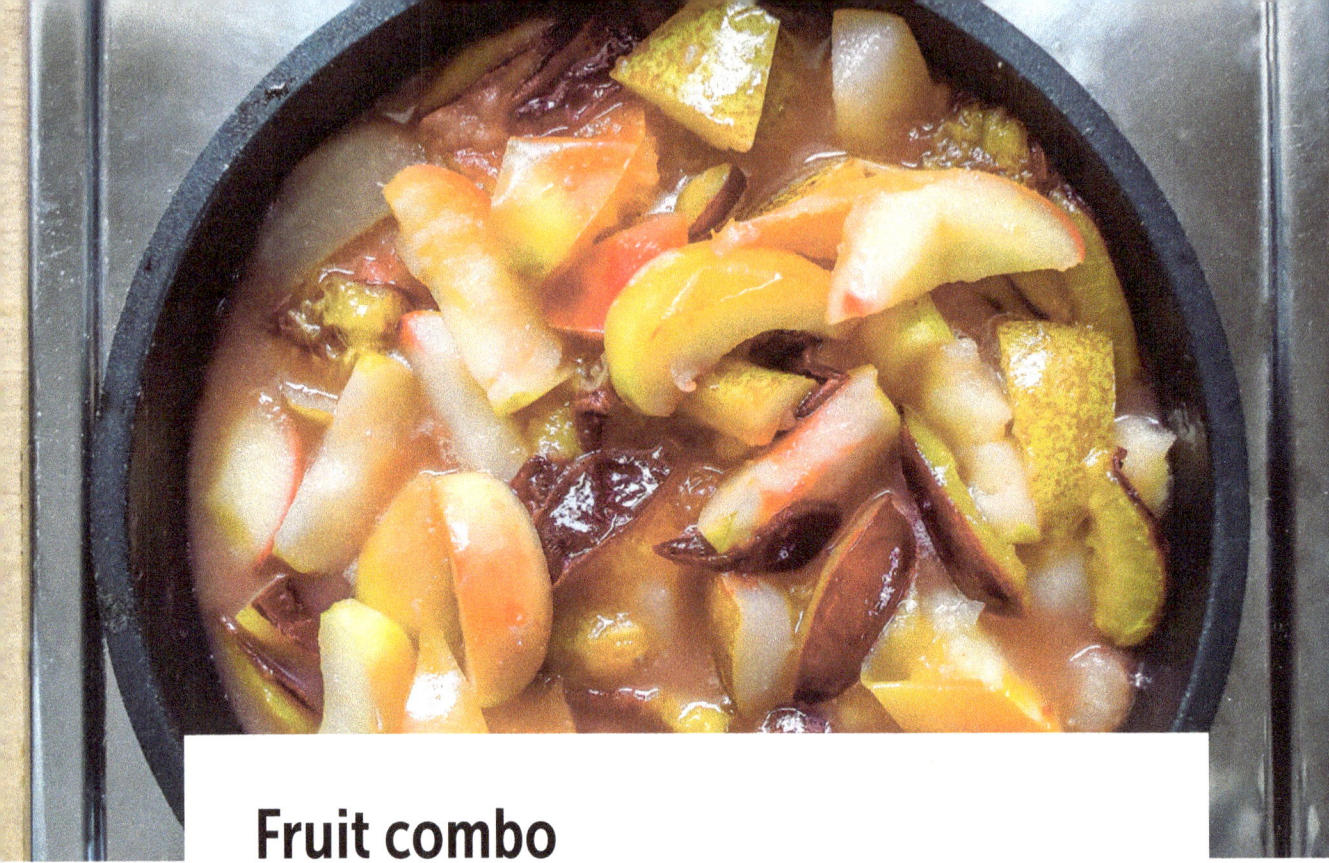

Fruit combo

If you enjoy apple crumble but can't be bothered making the topping, then this recipe is an easy one to try.

It is the type of dish that you could whip up in an instant if an unexpected guest arrives. If any fruit combo is left over, it is great for breakfast on the next day, hot or cold, served with cereal and yoghurt.

Ingredients

5 apples, peeled and sliced (or 1 x 500g (1lb) can sliced apple or pears)
130g (4½ oz) frozen berries
1 banana (optional)
10 dried apricots, slivered

1 lemon, juice and rind
2 Tbsp currants, sultanas or craisins
2 Tbsp almonds, slivered
½ tsp cinnamon

Method

1. Place all the ingredients into a bowl.
2. Microwave for 7–10 minutes on high.
3. Serve hot with yoghurt or sorbet.
4. For variation, replace berries with tamarillos or rhubarb. Stone fruit can also be used if in season; leave on the skin for more fibre as portrayed above.
5. This is great when reheated on the next day with cereal and yoghurt, or as a winter dessert.

Serves: 6.
Each serving contains: Energy 597kJ/142kcals; Protein 2g; Fat 3g; Saturated fat 0.4g; Carbohydrate 24g; Dietary fibre 5g; Sodium 4mg

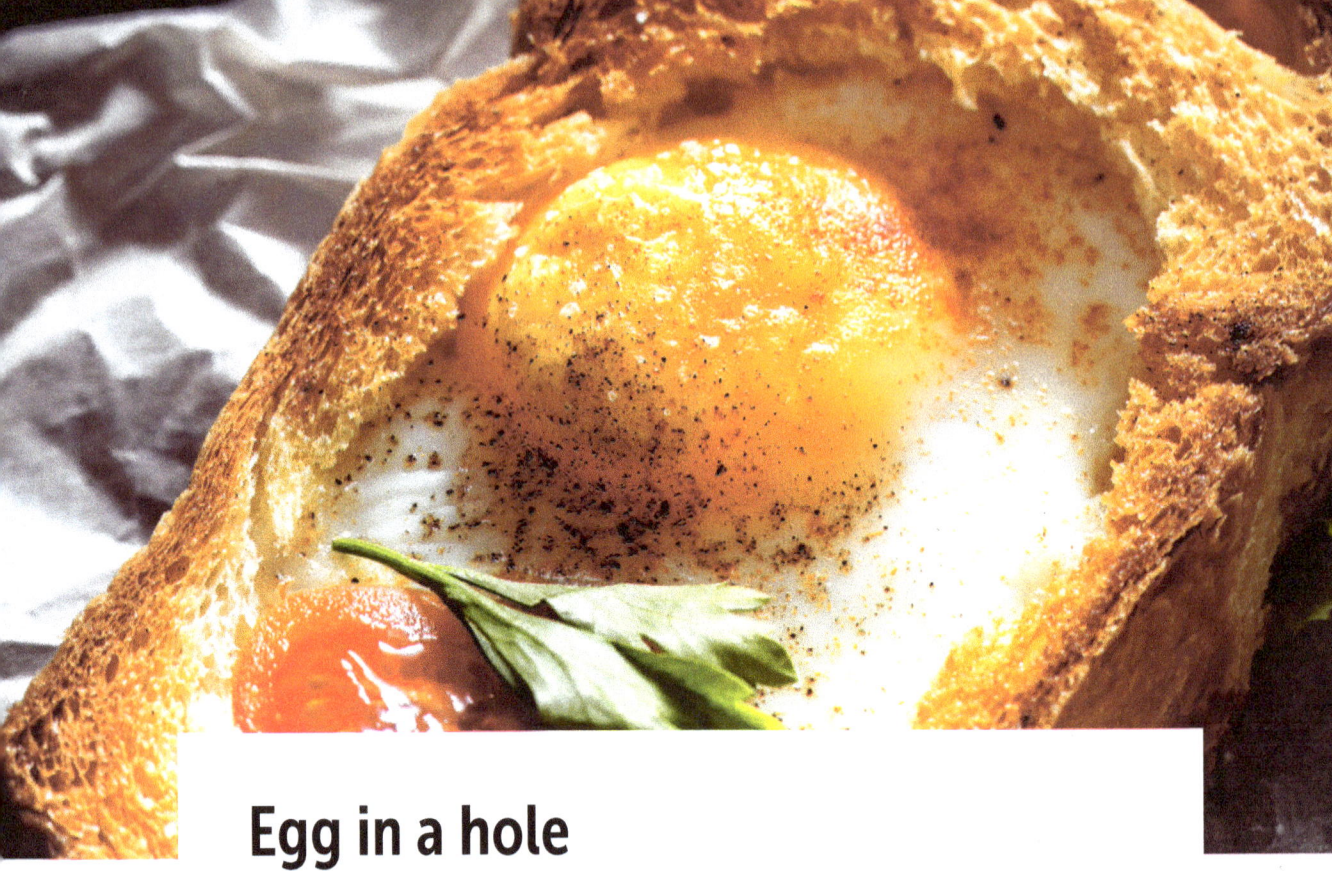

Egg in a hole

Without doubt, eggs are one of the cheapest forms of good quality protein in our diet today. They are rich in B group vitamins, Vitamin A and B12, and are perfectly safe to eat daily.

This recipe is easy to rustle up and fun for children to make for breakfast or lunch at weekends, or during school holidays.

Ingredients

1 wholegrain slice of bread
1 tsp margarine
1 egg, whole, raw

2 tsp spring onion, chopped
2 tsp tomato or red capsicum, finely chopped

Method

1. Spread the bread with margarine.
2. Using a cookie cutter or inverted glass, cut a hole in the middle of the

bread.

3. Heat a non-stick frypan on the stove to a temperature hot enough for a droplet of water to sizzle.
4. Place the bread margarine-side down into the pan; move the bread around so as to grease the pan beneath the hole.
5. Carefully break a raw egg into the hole in the bread.
6. Top with the spring onion and tomato.
7. Cover the pan with a lid.
8. Lower the heat of the pan slightly and cook until the egg appears cooked.
9. Using a fish slice, gently loosen the egg from the pan and flip over to cook the top.
10. When both sides are cooked, serve the egg on a warmed plate and enjoy.

Serves: 1.
Each serving contains: Energy 607kJ/145kcals; Protein 8.3g; Fat 7.4g; Saturated fat 1.9; Carbohydrate 11.5g; Dietary fibre 1.8g; Sodium 265mg

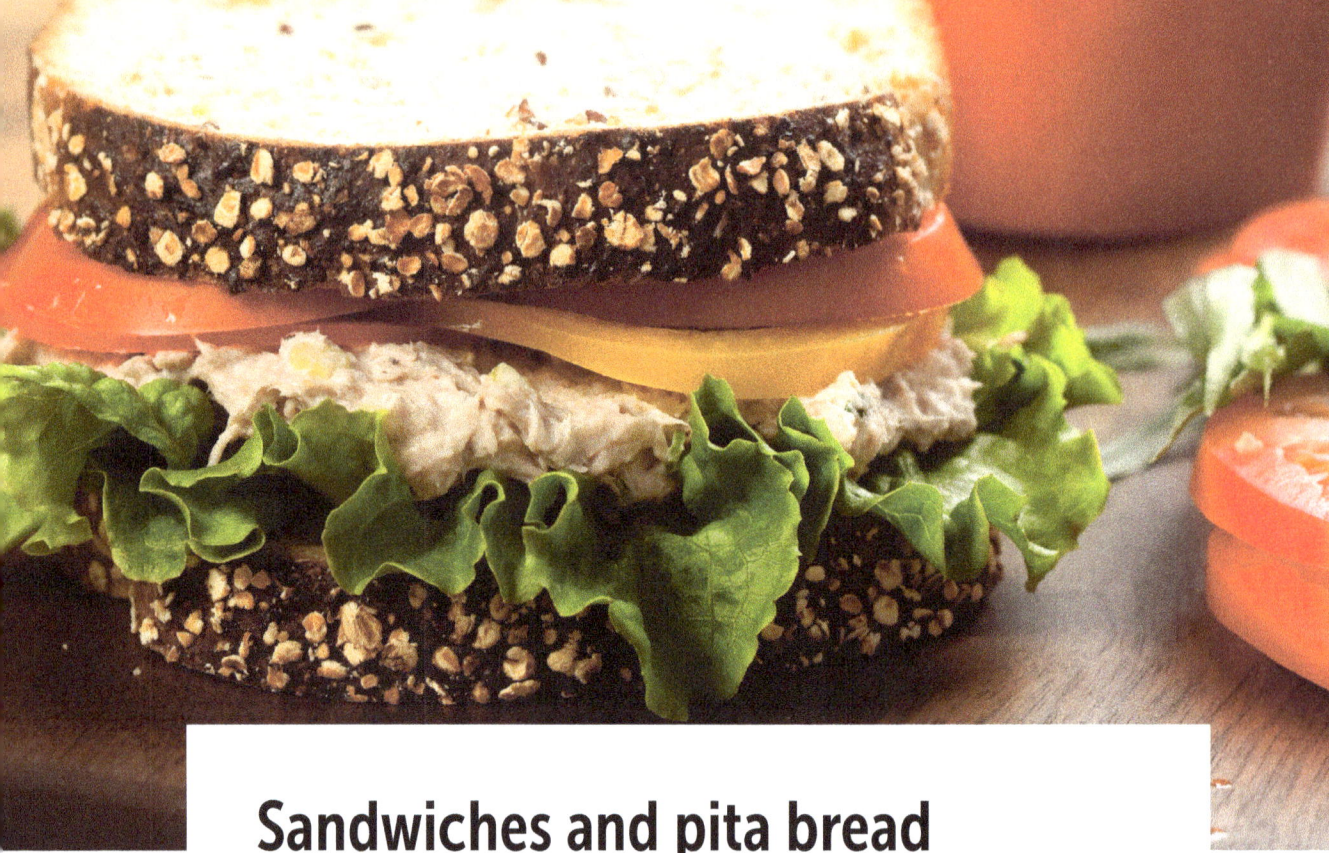

Sandwiches and pita bread

School lunches don't have to be boring but it is really important that they do get eaten, as they represent one-third of your child's daily intake.

With so many types of breads now on the market, such as wraps, paninis, pita bread, and bagels, lunches need never be dull. Try these combinations to make a great, tasty lunch!

Fillings

- Boiled egg with: chopped gherkin; grated carrot; green peas or corn
- Cottage cheese, chopped date, and dried apricot
- Grated carrot, raisins, chopped walnuts, and parsley
- Sliced orange, spring onion, lettuce, and sunflower seeds
- Cottage cheese, grated carrot, corn kernels, and sliced cucumber
- Cottage cheese, chopped mint, and drained crushed pineapple

- Peanut butter and salad vegetables
- Cottage cheese, chopped walnuts, raisins, and grated carrot
- Hummus and fresh salad vegetables
- Lettuce, tabbouleh, sliced capsicum, tomato, and red onion

To increase variety

- Vary the shape of sandwiches (e.g. pinwheel, club, or roll)
- Vary the colour and texture of bread
- Use the different grains (e.g. rye, cornbread, or French baguette)
- Combine white and brown bread into club sandwiches
- Buy rolls topped with cheese, poppy, or sesame seeds
- Roll slices of bread around asparagus, grated cheese and onion, cheese and pineapple, chicken pieces, minced ham

Make individual pie shells using leftover bread and fill with savoury combinations: cheese, corn, onion, ham or bacon, fish, tomato, mushroom, etc.

Pizzas and toasted sandwiches (filled with low-fat cheese; creamed corn or crushed pineapple or baked beans) are a meal in themselves, but are especially great for active children and growing teenagers playing sport after school.

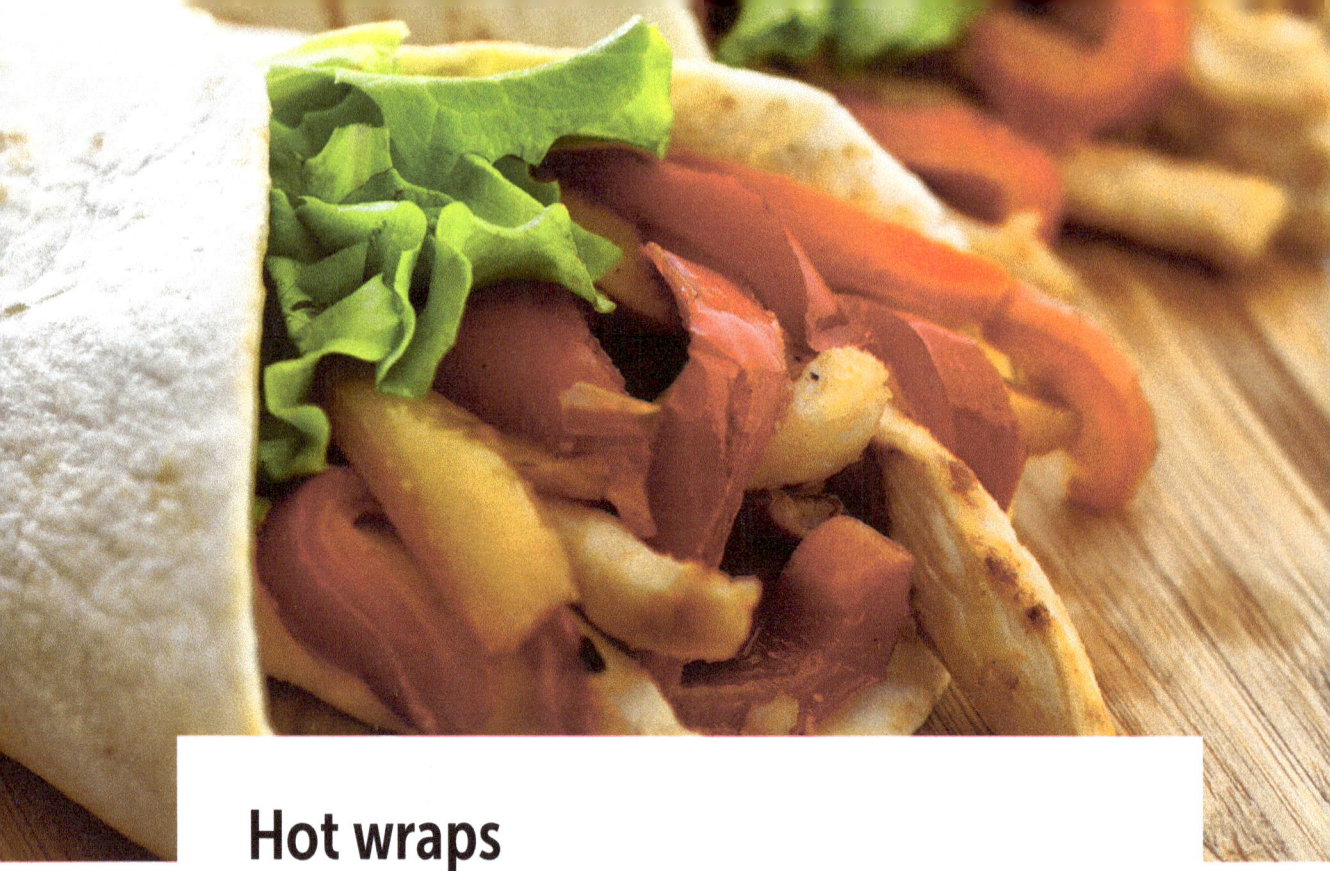

Hot wraps

Move over, sandwiches and rolls - wraps are here.

Pita pockets, tortillas and mountain bread all provide a quick way to bundle up food to eat. Cold or hot is fine, although if you are serving this as a hot main meal with a sauce over the top, then the thicker bread will be more sustaining. Also, these types of meals are an easy way to use up leftovers and represent them in a modern, fresh way.

Ingredients

45g (1½ oz) spinach, raw, chopped
3 button mushrooms, sliced
2 Tbsp red capsicum
1 wholegrain wrap

2 Tbsp Hummus
2 Tbsp cottage cheese
2 tsp Tuna or salmon or grated Edam cheese

Method

1. Place the spinach, mushrooms, and capsicum into a small microwave-safe dish; cover with cling film and microwave on high for 1.5 minutes.
2. Place the wrap onto a plate.
3. Spread the hummus over half the wrap, add the cottage cheese and fish (or grated cheese).
4. Then drain any juices from the hot vegetables and place these on top of the other wrap fillings.
5. Roll up the wrap; return to the microwave and reheat for 1.5 to 2 minutes.
6. Serve with salad plus your favourite relish or tomato sauce.
7. For a cold wrap you can substitute the spinach for lettuce, and the tuna for cooked chicken as portrayed above.

Serves: 1.
Each serving contains: Energy 1412kJ/337kcals; Protein 16g; Fat 17g; Saturated fat 2.8g; Carbohdyrate 29g; Dietary fibre 6.5g; Sodium 638mg

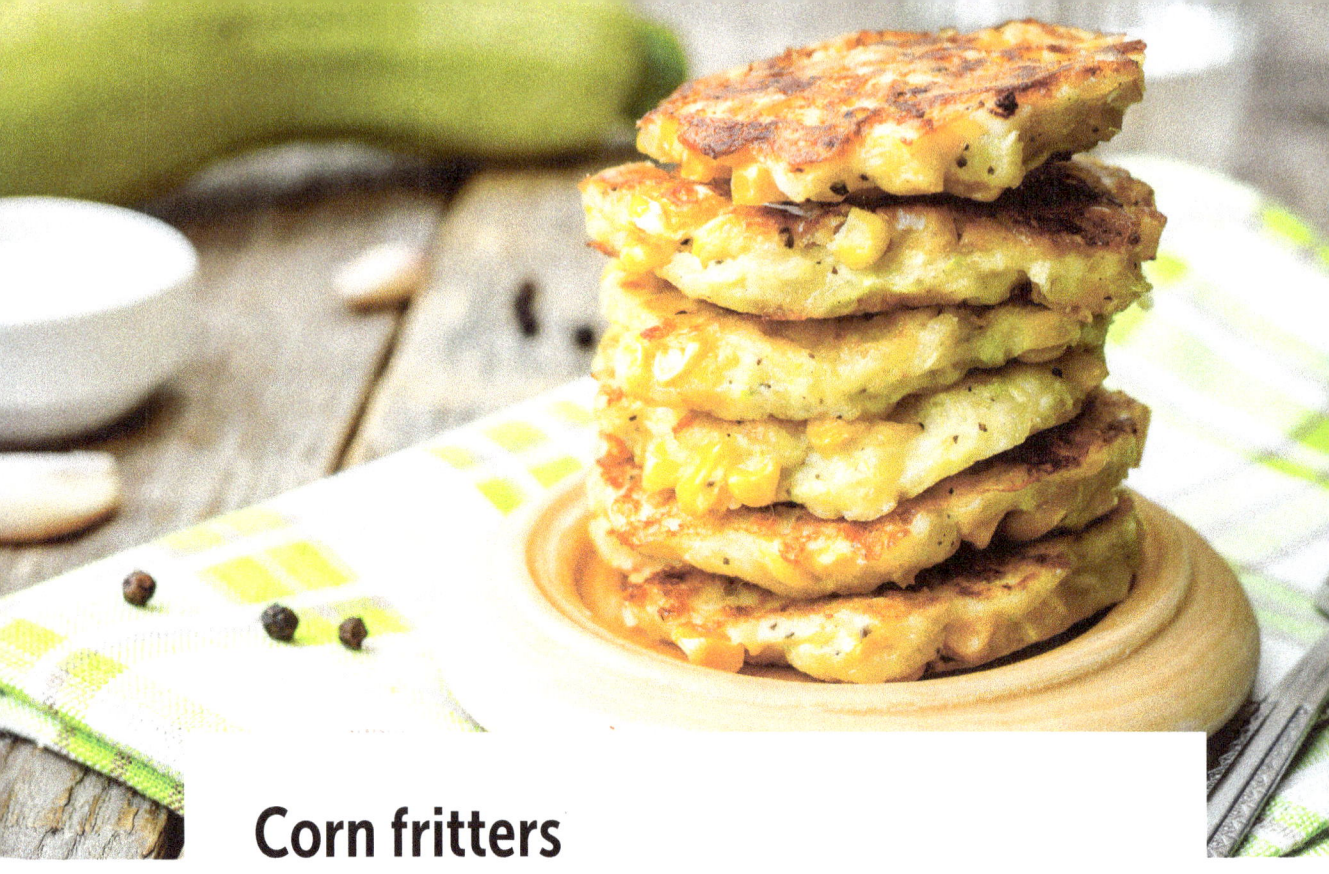

Corn fritters

Corn fritters are a cheap dish to serve if you have lots of people to feed and are so easy that children can make them during their school holidays.

Although this recipe uses corn, fritter batters can become the binding agent for lots of other ingredients such as fish, beans, leftover vegetables, or chopped cold cooked meat, so do try some of our suggested variations.

Ingredients

1 egg, beaten
250ml (8 fl oz) low-fat milk
125g (4 oz) plain white flour
2 tsp baking powder
410g (14½ oz) can sweet corn, drained

1 spring onion, finely chopped
3 Tbsp fresh parsley or coriander, chopped
2 Tbsp spicy tomato salsa, medium
½ tsp salt (optional)
1 Tbsp oil for cooking

Method

1. Turn on the warming drawer of your oven. Place a serving plate to warm while you make the fritters.
2. Break the egg into a medium-sized bowl; add the milk, and beat well.
3. Add to this mixture the flour, baking powder, salt, herbs, spring onion, and salsa. Using a fork, stir lightly to combine the ingredients.
4. Leave the mixture to rest for 1-2 minutes while you heat a moderately sized fry pan on the stove, adding 1 Tbsp of oil (per batch) just to lightly grease the pan. Use just enough oil to stop the fritters from sticking, not to deep fry.
5. When the oil begins to sizzle, add a dessert spoonful of mixture for each fritter. Cook in batches of 5-6 fritters at a time, depending on the size of your pan.
6. When you start to see bubbles rising in the mixture, carefully turn the fritters over using a fish slice.
7. Allow to cook until lightly brown, then transfer these cooked fritters to the dish in the warming drawer and return to making the next batch. Repeat this cooking process until all the mixture is used and you are ready to serve.

Serves: 6 (18 fritters)
Each fritter contains: Energy 295kJ / 70.5 kcal; Protein 2g; Fat 3g; Saturated fat 0.4g; Carbohydrate 9g; Dietary fibre 1g; Sodium 200mg

Variations

> Try varying the type of oil used in cooking, e.g. avocado (lime infused) or olive oil (infused with orange, lemon, or garlic).
> In place of corn, try chopped leftover lean meat; vegetables; or tuna.
> Vegetarians can boost the protein by adding tofu, chickpeas, or beans.
> These fritters can also be made very small for young children or served as party nibbles, with toothpicks and dipping sauces, or with fruit chutney or gucamole. Just mind the sodium.

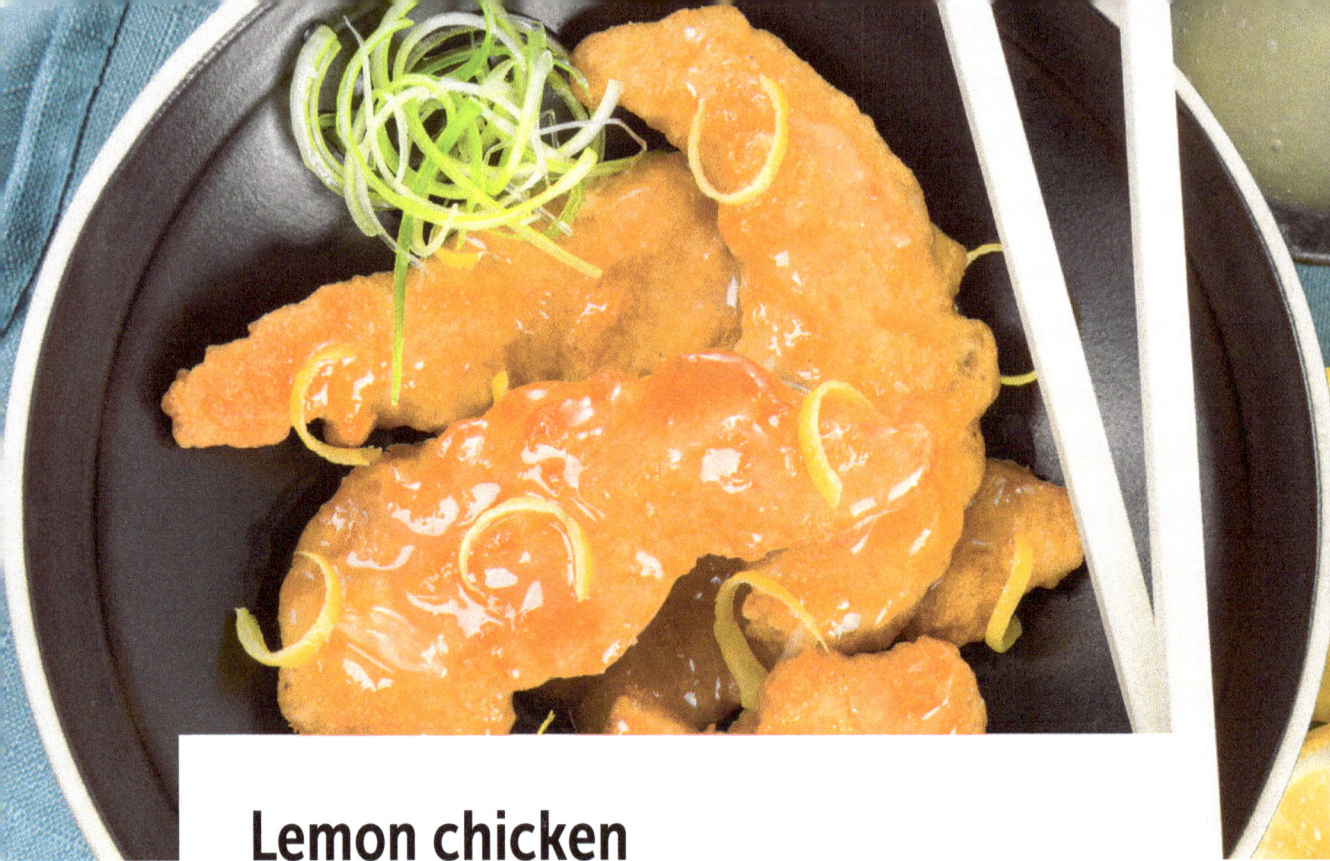

Lemon chicken

This recipe is a family favourite because it always works, has a terrific flavour, and is very forgiving if overcooked.

It can be served hot as a main dish, or is also great when left to chill, along with salad. The sauce forms a coating, making it ideal for picnics or cold buffet meals and when cut up, makes a great sandwich filling.

You might also like to give the same treatment to chicken wings or fish pieces and serve them cold, or warm as a party snack. The recipe is so easy a child could make it.

Ingredients

4 chicken breasts, skinned
Juice of 2 oranges, squeezed
Juice of 3 lemons, squeezed
3 Tbsp cornflour

1 Tbsp curry powder
2 Tbsp honey
1 Tbsp wholegrain mustard

Method

1. Skin the chicken and slice each breast into quarters.
2. Combine the curry and cornflour; toss the chicken pieces until well coated.
3. Place into a baking dish.
4. Make the sauce: squeeze the oranges and lemons into a glass jug, add the honey and mustard, and microwave on high for 2 minutes.
5. Pour the sauce over the chicken, and cover with foil.
6. Bake for 45-60 minutes on 180°C (350°F).
7. During the last 10-15 minutes of cooking, remove the foil so the chicken will brown.
8. Serve hot or cold with salad and vegetables, or alongside chop sticks and rice if wanting an Asian-style presentation as portrayed above.

Serves: 4.
Each serving contains: Energy 1429kJ/249kcals; Protein 28g; Carbohydrate 22g; Fat 4.6g; Dietary fibre 0.7g, Sodium 149mg

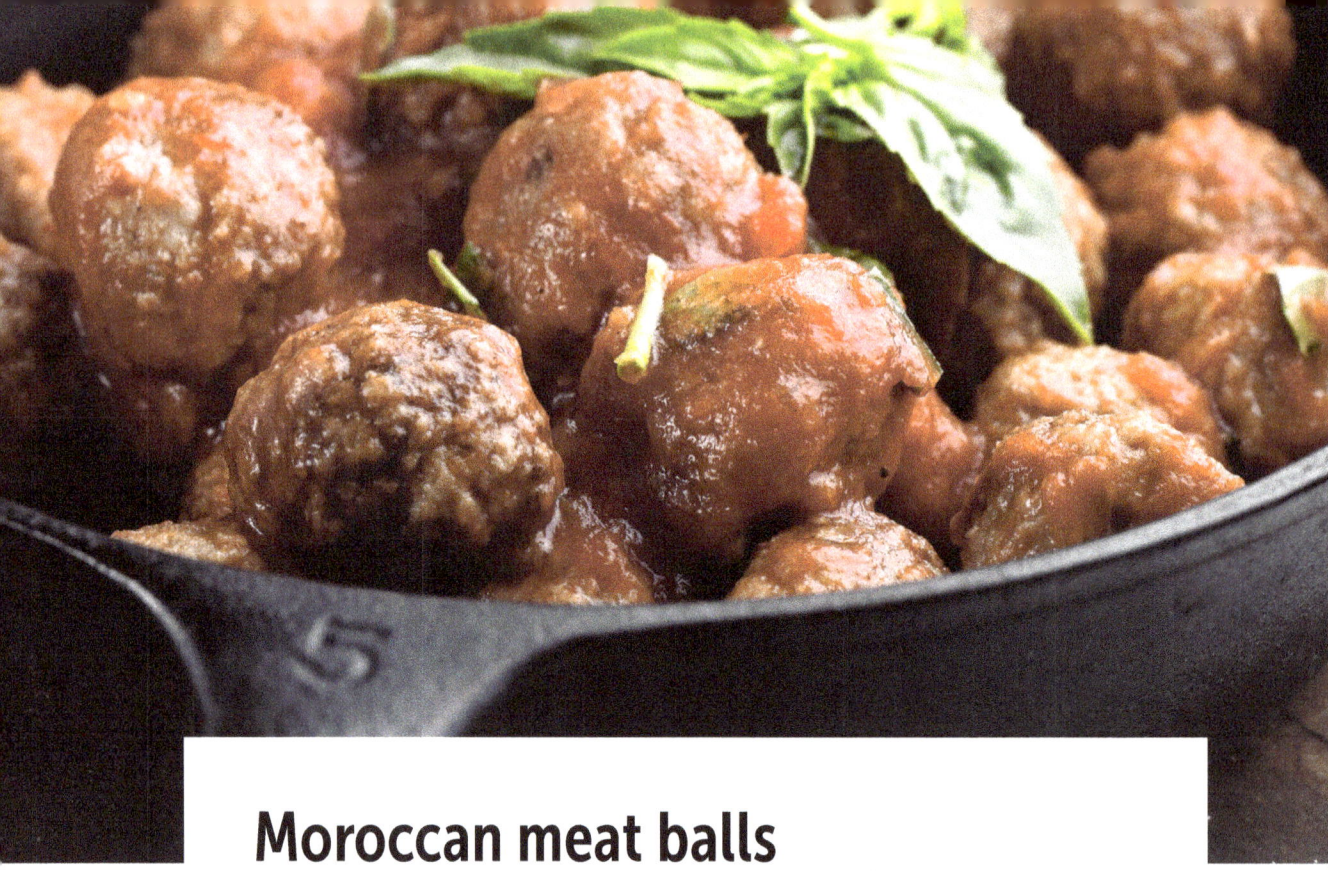

Moroccan meat balls

Meatballs are very versatile, and an easy way to encourage people to eat meat. Small enough to pop into the mouths of children or the elderly, they are a an excellent source of protein and iron.

As a main meal, meatballs can be served with a variety of sauces, with pasta or rice, or served dry for lunch or as a light meal. When added to salad, meatballs also provide a great filling in a pita pocket or panini, just the thing to fill hungry children as a lunchbox treat or an after-sport snack.

If you are entertaining, these meatballs can also be made smaller and served with toothpicks as a finger food alongside dipping sauces, such as sweet chilli or tzatziki.

Ingredients

500g (1 lb) lamb, minced
1 egg, lightly beaten
2 cloves garlic, crushed
1 tsp cumin
2 tsp paprika
3 Tbsp mint, chopped finely

2 Tbsp lemon juice
1 Tbsp lemon zest
2 Tbsp spicy tomato salsa, medium (optional)
3 Tbsp dry breadcrumbs (optional)
3 Tbsp olive oil

Method

1. Place the meat into a medium sized mixing bowl. Add the egg, garlic, cumin, paprika, mint, lemon juice and zest and salsa. Mix well
2. Using a dessert spoon, place small spoonfuls of mixture into the palm of your hand. Roll the spoonfuls and shape into small balls.
3. If you prefer your meatballs coated, then roll these in the breadcrumbs.
4. Heat the oil carefully in a non-stick frypan. When the pan is hot enough to make a drop of water sizzle, then add the meatballs. Keep shaking the pan to stop the balls from sticking. Using a metal and a wooden spoon, turn the balls carefully until they are all cooked.
5. You can serve onto a platter, or place on individual plates of pasta or rice, and then pour over a heated sauce.

Serves: 4–6 (24 balls)
Each ball contains: Energy 260kJ/62 Kcal; Protein 4.7g; Fat 4.5g; Saturated fat 1.3g; Carbohydrate 0.8g; Dietary Fibre negligible; Sodium 29mg

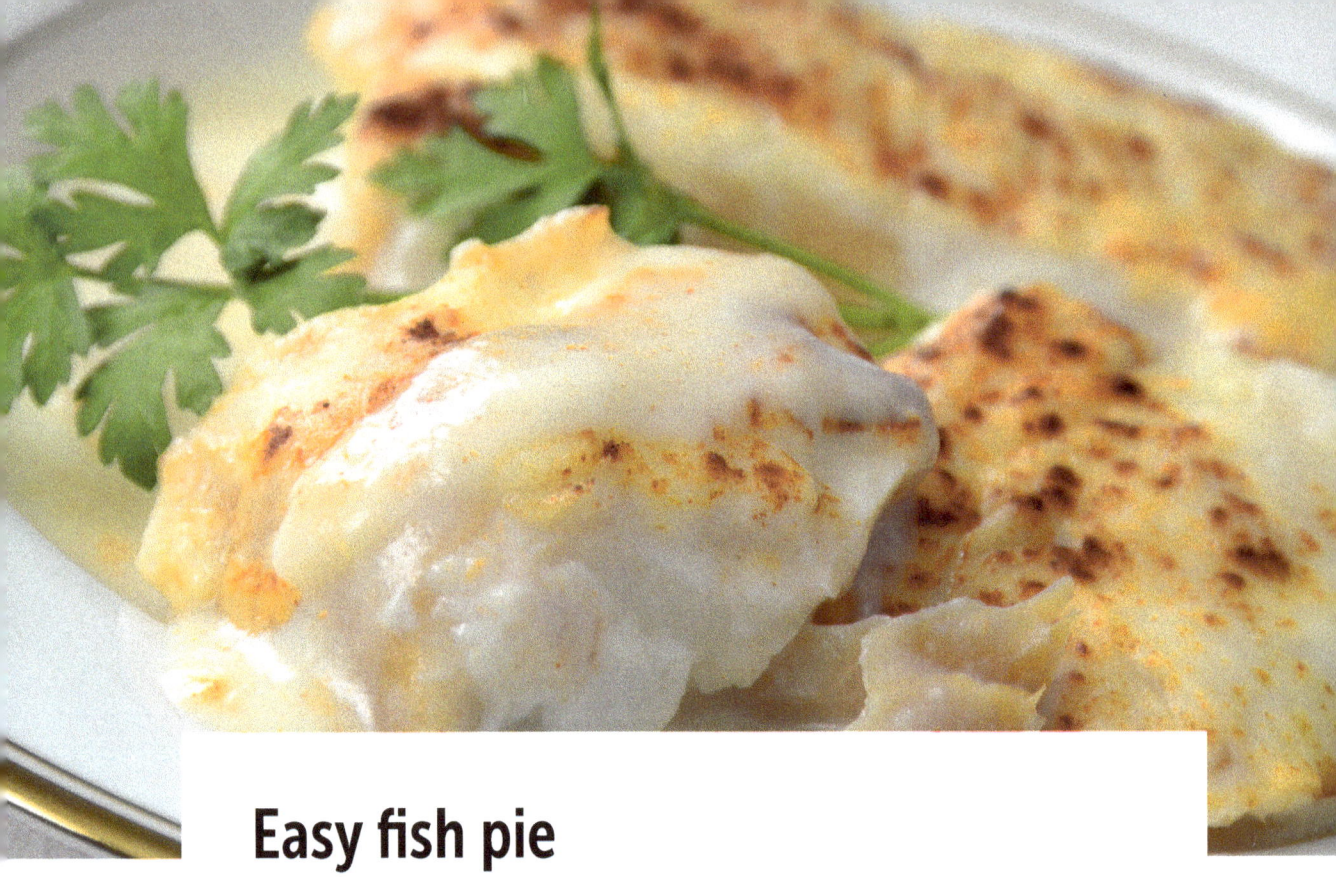

Easy fish pie

This fish dish is super easy to make, tastes amazing, and is easy to vary.

You can use any firm fish such as monkfish or gurnard. It also has the type of topping you could add to other meat dishes, such as chicken or veal, or use it for a speedy topping to vegetable bakes or lasagnas.

If you would like to lower the fat content even further, without spoiling the quality you can use half crème fraîche and half low-fat plain yoghurt, or ricotta cheese and lite sour cream.

Ingredients

600g (1 lb 5oz) fish fillets
60ml (2 fl oz) low-fat milk
250g (8½ oz) crème fraîche
60ml (2 fl oz) lemon juice
Rind of 2 lemons, coarsely grated

2 spring onions, finely chopped
1 Tbsp wholegrain mustard
1 Tbsp fresh coriander, chopped

Method

1. Place the fish into a shallow baking dish.
2. Add the low-fat milk.
3. Bake on 180°C (350°F) for 10–15 minutes or until the fish is lightly cooked.
4. In a small bowl, combine the crème fraîche, spring onions, lemon juice and rind, and the mustard.
5. Carefully drain off the excess milk and juices from the fish.
6. Top with the crème fraîche topping.
7. Grill the dish until the topping is lightly browned.
8. Sprinkle with chopped coriander.
9. Serve with vegetables or salad, rice, or mashed potato.

Serves: 4
Each serving contains: Energy 255kcal/1073kJ; Protein 28g; Fat 14g; Carbohydrate 3g; Dietary Fibre 1.6g; Sodium 225mg

Variations

> This dish does have a delicate flavour. For more spice, brush the fish (before adding milk) with your favourite chili and lime sauce, or add curry or cumin.

> For a more tropical, sweeter flavour, try adding either drained crushed pineapple or freshly sliced apricots or nectarines. (Note: This will increase the carbohydrate content.)

Additional recipes and resources

Recipes

Further healthy recipes (leastening.com/recipes) are available for family meals and snacks.

References

For an up-to-date list of references and further reading, please visit my website: http://www.leastening.com/references

Other Resources Available

The following organisations also have articles, food facts and recipes that may help you and your family find better health.

- Vegetables: www.vegetables.co.nz
- New Zealand Beef and Lamb: www.beeflambnz.co.nz
- NZ Vegetarian Society www.vegetarian.org.nz
- NZ Coeliac Society: www.coeliac.org.nz
- NZ Heart Foundation: www.heartfoundation.org.nz/resources/P12
- Diabetes NZ: www.diabetes.org.nz/home
- Dietitians NZ: http://dietitians.org.nz
- Dietitians Australia: https://daa.asn.au
- Sport NZ http://sportnz.org.nz
- Sleep Health Foundation Australia: www.sleephealthfoundation.org.au/public-information/fact-sheets-a-z/230-sleep-needs-across-the-lifespan.html
- Health Promotion Agency My Family Food myfamily.kiwi/foods
- Jamie's Food Revolution: Join Jamie's global movement to improve child nutrition www.jamiesfoodrevolution.org

Contact

Lea Stening
Dietitian and Nutrition Consultant
Christchurch, New Zealand
nutrition@leastening.com
www.leastening.com

About the author

Lea is a Dietitian with over 40 years' experience who works in private practice. She offers personal consultations online and also provides nutrition seminars to sporting, school, workplace, and community groups.

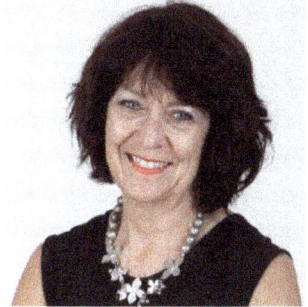

Lea's work has taken her overseas to Melbourne and London where she has worked in hospitals and private clinics, helping people with dietary-related health problems such as diabetes, cancer, heart disease, gastro-intestinal problems, allergies and intolerances, etc.

Specialising in Sports nutrition and Paediatrics, Lea is passionate about helping developing athletes and their families improve their performance through better nutrition. Lea has worked in all school sports also nationally at High Performance and Academy levels for 8 years in cricket, 5 years in rowing, and 12 years in Paralympian sports.

Health promotion has also been an important part of Lea's work, involving public lectures, writing regular newspaper and magazine articles, as well as conducting televison and radio interviews.

As a Food Revolution Ambassador for New Zealand, Lea believes that all food educators, working together globally, can improve the health and education outcomes of our children through better nutrition, love, and care.

Other books by the author
Nutrition Manual for Developing Rowers, 2005
From Playground to Podium, late 2017

Acknowledgements

Thank you to all the parents, throughout my career, whose experiences feeding their children have contributed to the direction of this book.

Also special thanks to my family for their love and support, particularly to my son Jonathan for his design and technical assistance.

www.ingramcontent.com/pod-product-compliance
Lightning Source LLC
Chambersburg PA
CBHW061749290426
44108CB00028B/2939